Biotanical Health   USA: 1-800- 893-031

MW01222250

BIOTANICAL HEALTH

PRODUCT MANUAL

August 2008

Please put your herbs in the refrigerator to maintain their freshness and potency.

Biotanical Health   USA: 1-800- 893-0319   UK: 020-8133-9730

Published by Biotanical Health

14525 SW Millikan Way, Beaverton, OR 97005-2343, USA

1-732-333-1868

This book is not intended to take the place of medical advice from a trained medical professional. Readers are advised to consult a physician or other qualified health professional regarding treatment of their medical problems.

Please consult a physician or other qualified health professional before attempting any natural health or cleansing programs.

ISBN 1440403090

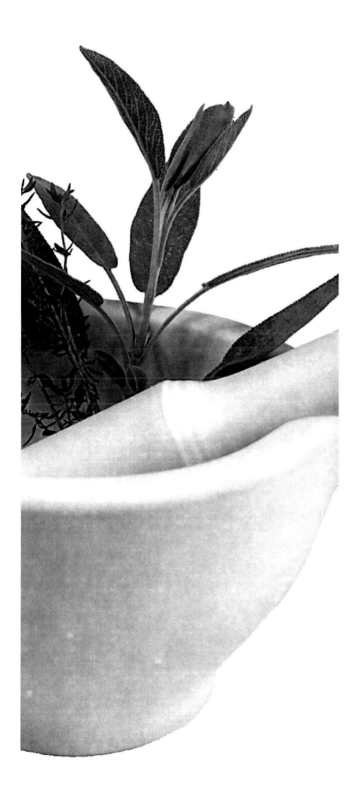

Contents

WHY MY HERBS WORK

My herbal blends are stronger because I use only organic and wild-crafted herbs. The herbs I source have been grown in nutrient-dense soil, under optimal conditions, giving them 3 to 9 times more potency than regular herbs.

My herbs are 100% pure. Unlike the herbs you can get on websites and health food stores, mine are not sprayed with pesticides and fertilizers. They are not irradiated or chemically treated in any way.

My herbs have been tried and tested on my own personal client base. I actually make most of my income from private consultations with clients, not from selling herbs. If my herbal blends were not effective, I would not get repeat consultations and referrals.

My herbal blends are based on scientific research, and what's been working for thousands of years in Traditional Chinese Medicine. I have hundreds of happy clients who have benefited from taking herbal blends that work.

Amina Christy

Welcome

Congratulations on making the wise decision to purchase a natural organic remedy!

Welcome to Biotanical Health's new-style Product Manual, incorporating instructions for using our products. We have had many requests for "offline" information and are pleased to provide this manual to you in order to show you how to get the most from your herbal remedies.. We hope you find it useful.

All our herbal formulations have been designed to help you achieve your health goals in the shortest period of time – whether your objective is to lose weight, improve your energy levels, fertility or reproductive health, we aim to provide you with the best quality organic and wildcrafted herbal remedies.

Please Put Your Herbal Remedies In The Refrigerator

Because our herbal remedies do not contain any artificial preservatives, they will need to be stored in the refrigerator to maintain their potency and freshness.

How To Contact Us

For the fastest possible service, please email one of our Customer Service Assistants, who will be able to assist you with any questions you have about our products.

You can contact them via email: orders@biotanicalhealth.com or by leaving a telephone message at: 1-732-333-1868 (This is a USA phone number). Your message will be transcribed and emailed to Customer Services, so please leave a valid email address, so that you will get a prompt response.

How To Order Herbal Remedies

You can order online via our website: www.biotanicalhealth.com Or order via telephone:

USA. 1-800- 893-0319

UK: 020-8133-9730

Press 1 only if you are ready to order, so that you will be forwarded to our Order Processing Center.

Share Your Success Story!

We have included a few of our most recent success stories in this book, to demonstrate how people just like you are benefitting from our natural herbal remedies.

If you have a story you'd like to share with everyone, please contact us via:

www.BiotanicalCustomers.com

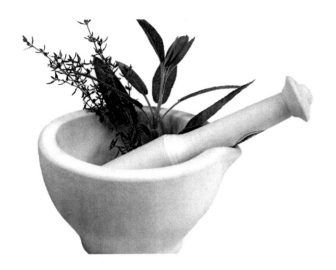

A detoxification program, combined with a healthy diet and herbal remedies can assist your organs in healing themselves, restore the metabolic rate, improve reproductive health, and improve the body's immunity to disease and chronic conditions.

Body Cleansing

Body Cleansing is the foundation of any natural health program. Detoxification programs that remove built up toxins can improve the functioning and the efficiency of the organs of elimination, helping the body to heal itself naturally, and allowing for a greater absorption of the nutrients in your food. Best of all… body cleansing makes your herbal remedies twice as effective.

Benefits of Body Cleansing

The need to cleanse and detoxify the body has become increasingly more important over the past 50 years. This is because the chemical industry has introduced many new and dangerous chemical toxins and byproducts into our soil, water supply, and into the air that we breathe. It's impossible to avoid these toxins as they are everywhere. For example there are over 75,000 synthetic chemicals registered with the U.S. Environmental Protection Agency, and this does not even include the chemicals produced in other parts of the world.

The chemical industry releases over 24 billion pounds of toxic chemicals are released into the environment, and the long-term effects of those chemicals, or whether they interact dangerously with each other is currently unknown. Is it any wonder that every Western society is experiencing an increase in chronic and degenerative diseases? Even though billions of dollars are invested in medical research, the Center For Disease Control still estimates that 1 out of 2 men and 1 out of 3 women will be diagnosed with cancer in their lifetime.

It has only been as recent as 2003 that the medical establishment have recognized there is a link between disease and these toxic chemicals. A 2003 study conducted by the Mt. Sinai School of Medicine found an average of 91 of these chemicals in a group of subjects, which included people who had eaten organic foods for over 25 years.

The Effects Of These Chemicals

It's not just environmental pollutants we need to be aware of. These chemicals have also made their way into our food, in the form of artificial preservatives, flavorings, colorings and other types of additives. In addition to this, non-organic forms of meat and dairy have been contaminated by growth hormones, antibiotics and drugs fed to livestock to increase their weight (and selling price.)

It is not surprising then that every cell, organ and system of our body is affected by these chemical toxins. For example, toxins in the nervous system cause depression, irritability and an inability to cope with life's challengers. In the digestive system, they cause a wide range of symptoms, including Irritable Bowel Syndrome, constipation, diarrhea and even recurrent headaches.

More recently, scientists have linked these toxins to reproductive complaints such as unexplained infertility, fibroids, Polycystic Ovarian Syndrome, endometriosis, low sperm counts, poor motility and morphology, and a lack of sex drive in both men and women. They even affect our immune systems, which make us vulnerable to yeast infections, Pelvic Inflammatory Disease, and chlamydia – both of which are common causes of blocked fallopian tubes in women.

These chemicals even affect our weight. This is because a toxic digestive system and liver will slow down the metabolic rate, causing the body to convert more energy into body fat. Low energy levels brought on by excessive toxins mean that exercise becomes increasingly difficult, leading to a loss in muscle tissue, and a further decrease in metabolic rate. It is also well-known among natural healers that toxins stored in fat are more resistant to diet and exercise.

This is why a detoxification program, combined with a healthy diet and herbal remedies can assist your organs in healing themselves, restore the metabolic rate, improve reproductive health, and improve the body's immunity to disease and chronic conditions.

Body Cleansing Schedule

The 28-day body cleansing program allows you to to cleanse your body without fasting. It is very gentle and can be combined with any of our herbal remedies.

Body Cleansing Schedule

Week	Cleansing Program	Products
Week 1	Colon Cleanse	Colon D-Tox 1 Colon D-Tox 2
Week 2	Liver & Gallbladder Cleanse	Liver D-Tox Tea Liver D-Tox Capsules
Week 3	Kidney & Bladder Cleanse	Kidney D-Tox Tea Kidney D-Tox Capsules
Week 4	Toxin Cleanse	Para D-Tox Metal D-Tox

How To Do A Body Cleanse

To achieve the best possible benefits while doing your cleanse, please follow the steps in the order given below:

1. Colon cleansing

2. Liver cleansing

3. Kidney cleansing

4. Toxin cleansing

The most convenient way to start the cleansing program is by starting on a Monday and performing each cleanse Monday to Friday, giving yourself the weekends to relax and prepare for your next cleanse.

If you are taking herbal remedies, e.g. for fertility, menstrual problems or weight loss, I recommend you take them alongside the cleanses. Generally, people start to see noticeable results after the cleanse phase is complete, as the body is better able to absorb and process the herbal remedies.

Do not do the cleanses all at once, as you will detoxify too quickly and overload your system. Follow the steps above for a gentle, symptom-free cleanse.

We recommend you take AlkaGreens Plus alongside your cleanse, to provide your body with additional nutrients required to support the organs during the cleanse, and to give you additional energy without adding many calories.

Frequently Asked Questions

Question: Can I Take Herbal Remedies While Cleansing?

Answer: Yes! Cleansing increases the effectiveness of your herbal remedies, and can give you faster, and longer-lasting results.

Question: Should I continue with the cleansing program if I become pregnant half way through?

Answer: No. If you become pregnant before completing the cleanse, do not continue the cleansing program. Focus on having a healthy pregnancy by taking AlkaGreens Plus with a good diet.

Customer Services will be happy to send you a free 1-month supply for sharing your success story.

Question: Will I experience a healing crisis?

Answer: A healing crisis happens when you detox too quickly and is characterized by headaches, tiredness, bloating, furry tongue, and skin complaints. The 4-week cleansing program is gentle enough to release toxins at a slower rate, so you will avoid experiencing these symptoms.

If you are very sensitive, consider supplementing your cleanse with AlkaGreens Plus, as it contains ingredients that bind to toxins and enable them to exit the body safely, without symptoms.

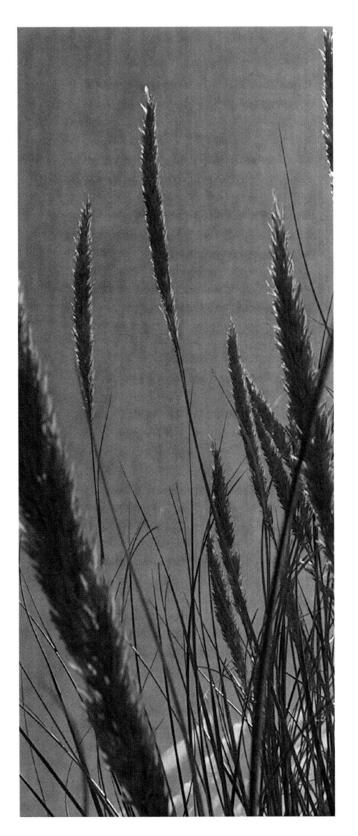

The first step in any cleansing program is to cleanse your colon and clear a path for all the toxins you are going to expel during the cleanse. Colon cleansing also improves the digestion, enabling you to absorb the nutrients in your food, and improve your health.

Colon Cleansing

A healthy colon is vital to maintaining good health. It's one of the major organs of elimination, and breaks down the toxins in our food and eliminates them as waste, but in order for this to occur, we should ideally have a bowel movement for every large meal that we eat. Yet most of us don't, and this is the cause of many illnesses facing people in modern times.

Many nutritionists, herbalists and alternative health practitioners believe that illnesses, including depression, skin problems, fatigue, reproductive challenges and even obesity have greatly increased in recent years due to putrefied wastes that accumulate in the colon and are reabsorbed by the body. Even healthy, nutritious food will begin to rot inside of our warm, moist bodies if it sits there long enough. Harmful bacteria will begin to grow., and healthy levels of beneficial bacteria will decrease in response.

It makes sense if you think about it. The longer a meal remains in our digestive tract, the longer we're exposed to the toxic, potentially carcinogenic substances that it contains, or will develop as it rots inside of your intestines.

While some of us have only one bowel movement a day, and others have just one a week, that's clearly too much solid waste for the colon to hold at one time. this is why diseases such as colon cancer, diverticulitis, diverticulosis, colitis and colon polyps are on the rise.

Although many types of pollution, stress, and a chronic lack of exercise can all contribute to a sluggish, poorly-eliminating colon, the main cause of our poor bowel habits is undoubtedly our diet. The modern diet now includes plenty of high-fat, high-sugar processed foods with little fiber or nutrients.

Your colon was not meant to process artificial chemical-ridden foods with little nutritional value, so ingesting them merely increases its workload with no discernible benefit. Processing large amounts of fat and proten is especially difficult, and a lack of fiber keeps food from moving through your digestive tract quickly and efficiently.

As a result, constipation has become so common that many rely on laxatives to "move things along". Unfortunately, laxatives can become habit-forming, so long-term users often become even more constipated when they stop using them! Laxative use also does nothing to address the underlying problem, and many laxatives contain chemicals that make the colon worse in the long term.

FACT: Did you know that Colon D-Tox 1 can help with constipation?

Benefits of Colon Cleansing

By completing an efficient colon cleanse at the beginning of your detoxification journey, you'll enjoy the following benefits:

- Relief from the symptoms of many digestive disorders, including irritable bowel syndrome, constipation and hemorrhoids

- Increased absorption of any vitamins, minerals, and other nutrients that you ingest

- Increased effectiveness of all other detoxification processes

- Reduction and/or elimination of intestinal parasites and their accompanying symptoms, including insomnia, diarrhea, nervousness, chronic pain, menstrual irregularities, and chronic fatigue

- Reduction and/or elimination of an overgrowth of Candida albicans, the yeast responsible for recurrent yeast infections, fungal infections like athlete's foot, and a host of other symptoms, from sugar cravings to chronic fatigue

- Strengthening of the colon wall, which will speed digestion and allow wastes to pass through the body more efficiently

- Creating an environment that will encourage healthy levels of friendly intestinal flora, which are necessary to maintaining balance in the colon

- Getting rid of excess intestinal gas and bloating, and reducing inflammation, giving you a flatter-looking abdomen.

Most people are shocked by the improvement that they feel after a successful colon cleanse lasting only five days!

	Colon Cleansing Schedule
Day 1	1 Capsule of Colon D-Tox 1 1 Spoon of Colon D-Tox 2
Day 2	2 Capsules of Colon D-Tox 1 2 Spoons of Colon D-Tox 2
Day 3	3 Capsules of Colon D-Tox 1 3 Spoons of Colon D-Tox 2
Day 4	4 Capsules of Colon D-Tox 1 4 Spoons of Colon D-Tox 2
Day 5	5 Capsules of Colon D-Tox 1 5 Spoons of Colon D-Tox 2

How To Do A Colon Cleanse

There are two steps to doing an effective colon cleanse. These steps are:

- Regulating the colon

- Detoxifying the colon

Regulating the colon

Before cleansing the colon, it's important to get it to work more effectively, so it can expel toxins. Regulating the colon involves taking herbs that gently stimulate the colon to expel waste more regularly. These herbs contain active compounds that stimulate the peristaltic action - this is the natural involuntary movement your intestines go through when passing food through its system.

Herbs that regulate the colon soothe its lining with mucus, allowing waste products to flow painlessly and easily through the colon. These include:

- African Bird Pepper – stimulates peristalsis, reduces cramping and intestinal gas and has a detoxifying effect

- Barberry Root Bark – kills harmful bacteria and improves the condition of the tissues of the digestive tract

- Cape Aloes – stimulates the colon, relieves constipation and accelerates healing of the tissues and mucus membranes of the colon

- Cascara Sagrada Aged Bark – softens stools and triggers peristalsis, the natural movement of the colon that moves food throughout the digestive system

- Fennel Seed – reduces inflammation, bloating and excess intestinal gas, and relieves intestinal spasms

- Garlic Bulb – a powerful detoxification agent that kills intestinal parasites, infection and harmful bacteria, helping to restore healthy fauna to the digestive system

- Ginger Root – destroys viruses, relieves pain and inflammation and controls nausea

- Senna Herb – stimulates peristaltic action and softens stools to clear the bowels painlessly

The Colon D-Tox Formula 1 contains the ingredients listed, and regulates the colon by stimulating peristaltic action, (this is the natural muscular contraction of your colon) reducing inflammation, bloating and gas, while removing harmful bacteria, to enable stools to pass through easily and painlessly.

To regulate your colon, start by taking one capsule of Colon D-Tox Formula 1 each day, with your evening meal, increasing your dose by one capsule each day, until your bowel movements become regular. The gradual increase is to avoid overdosing, which has the effect of loosening the bowels and increasing the frequency of defecation. Ideally, you should be moving your bowels 2-3 times a day.

Detoxifying the colon

Detoxifying the colon involves taking natural herbs and substances that soothe the colon, while creating an adhesive layer that draws out impacted waste from the colon walls.   Colon detoxification formulas are powerful enough to reach pockets within the colon, and ease out waste that could be causing inflammation, IBS or other bowel problems.

Typical ingredients in a Colon Detoxification Formula include:

- Activated Willow charcoal – absorbs artificial additives, toxins, gasses and chemicals from the colon walls, and binds them safely to be expelled by the colon

- Apple Fruit Pectin – contains enzymes that break down built up intestinal waste, and binds to toxic heavy metals, so they can be safely removed by the colon

- Flax Seeds – a rich source of fiber that bulks up the colon, strengthening the muscles of peristalsis, and allows waste to be carried out of the body quickly

- Marshmallow Root –reduces inflammation of the tissues of the intestinal tract, relieves indigestion and stimulates wound healing

- Peppermint Leaf – relieves indigestion, relaxes muscle spasms, reduces intestinal gas and soothes the tissues of the digestive tract

- Pharmaceutical Grade Bentonite Clay – absorbs and binds to encrusted fecal matter, absorbs toxins such as heavy metals, pesticides, viruses and molds

- Psyllium Seeds and Husks – relieves constipation and binds to intestinal waste. Increases bulk, enabling the waste to be expelled by the colon

- Slippery Elm Inner Bark – coats the tissues of the intestinal tract with a slippery mucus material, which has a soothing and lubricating effect, allowing for painless defecation

The Colon D-Tox Formula 2 helps to detoxify the colon by adhering itself to the impacted waste, so that it can be easily removed by the actions of the Colon D-Tox Formula 2.

Its ingredients are powerful enough to draw out toxic chemicals, drug residues, and harmful bacteria from the colon, while preserving the "good bacteria" in the colon that helps the digestive process.

It's very easy to take. Simply put one teaspoon of Colon D-Tox Formula 2 into a jar or bottle with 8oz (250 ml) of fruit juice or water. Shake the mixture vigorously and drink. Because Colon D-Tox Formula 2 is a natural bulk and fiber formula, you will need to drink at least 8oz (250 ml) of water after consuming the mixture.

To avoid lumps, you can mix the powder into a thick paste with a small amount of liquid, then keep adding more liquid until the mixture becomes runny. this takes a little longer to prepare than shaking, but gives a smoother drink.

For a more powerful colon cleansing effect, increase your intake of Colon D-Tox Formula 2 by one teaspoon a day.

Frequently Asked Questions

Question: How can I tell if it's working?

Answer: If you are following the directions given in this book, you should notice that your bowel movements become more regular after the first few days. they will also become softer and larger in volume.

Question: What If My Bowels Are Not Regular By The End Of The 5 Days?

Answer: If your bowels are very sluggish and you are only having one movement a day (but are eating 2-3 means a day, continue with the colon cleanse for another week, gradually increasing your dose of Colon D-Tox 1 until you are moving your bowels 2-3 times a day.

Colon D-Tox 1 is completely safe to take, so don't worry about taking too much. One client needed to take 40 capsules a day before his bowel movements were regular!

You will not have to increase your intake of Colon D-Tox 2 beyond 5 teaspoons a day.

Question: Can I still do the colon cleanse if I have colitis, crohn's disease or irritable bowel syndrome?

Answer: If you are prone to diarrhea, or any of the conditions above, skip Colon D-Tox 1 and use Colon D-Tox 2 on its own. Its ingredients can reduce inflammation and calm the irritated tissues of the colon.

Colon D-Tox 2 can also help relieve the symptoms of mild food poisoning, as its absorbent ingredients can soak up the poisons so they do less damage to your body. It also helps to make excessively loose bowel movements firmer.

Success Story

"My father was visiting me for two weeks and his visit happened to coincide with the start of my cleansing program.

We did the colon cleanse together and ate a healthy vegetarian diet, which included a lot of stir fries, Thai food, gourmet soups, a few out door picnics and some interesting rice and bean dishes.

For as long as I can remember, my father has always had a large belly for his height, but at the end of the 5 days, he was having to do his belt up 2 notches tighter!

He decided to continue with the colon cleanse, as he found it very beneficial. He was moving his bowels more regularly, said he felt a lot lighter, and had more energy to go sight-seeing, and enjoy the London night life!

By the time he was ready to go back home, we had to buy him a new pair of trousers, belt and underwear because he ha lost so much weight (5 inches from his belly)

My mother called me a few days later to ask what I had done to him, because he was now eating less, taking daily walks, and asking for vegetables with his meals!"

Yinka Adewole, London UK

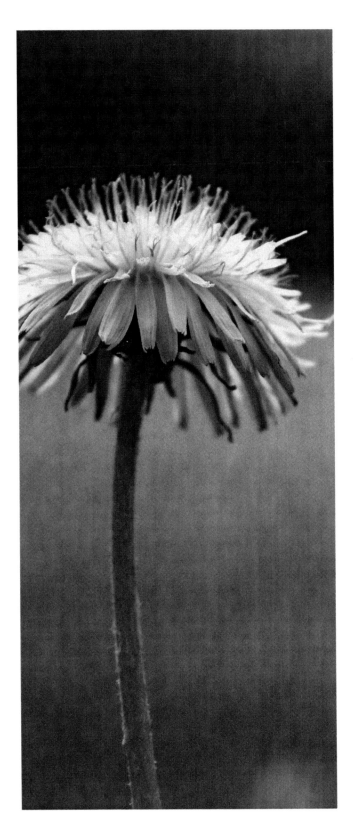

Everything you eat, drink, breathe or absorb through the skin is processed by the liver. Given that it is one of the largest organs in the body and is responsible for over 200 different processes, it's no wonder that livers can become congested! Many people report feeling energized after doing a liver cleanse, and you can cleanse your liver too, following these simple instructions,

Liver and Gallbladder Cleansing

The liver cleanse is an important cleanse for improving general health, as its primary role is to cleanse and detoxify the blood. Since everything you eat, drink, breathe or absorb through the skin eventually enters the bloodstream, the liver has a continuous job of filtering toxicity from the blood, in order to protect the organs.

The liver's main job is to break down old red blood cells, synthesize plasma proteins, produce bile to digest fats, store glycogen, a short term fuel. It is also responsible for breaking down hormones, such as estrogen and progesterone. In Traditional Chinese Medicine, the liver is a primary organ for fertility, as it the organ that helps to transform food into energy for every day activity as well as reproduction.

Modern living exposes us to more toxins than the liver can easily handle. Saturated fats, cholesterol, pharmaceutical drug residues, artificial additives, pesticides, preservatives, colorings, chemicals from our cleaning products and cosmetics, cigarette smoke, smog and artificial meat hormones all end up being broken down by the liver for elimination.

Although the liver is a regenerating organ, the exposure to harmful chemicals kills liver cells faster than the liver can regenerate them, resulting in a smaller and considerably weaker liver. The end result is a liver that cannot cope with the toxins taken in by the body, and the toxins being circulated to the organs via the blood, weakening our most vulnerable organs and causing harm and irritation to our cells.

A healthy liver should be your first line of defense against environmental and food toxins, because it should filter out these toxins and chemically neutralize them before they get circulated to the rest of your blood stream.

The gallbladder is responsible for storing bile, a liver byproduct that is used to neutralize toxins, break down dietary fats, stimulate the digestive process and trigger peristalsis. The gallbladder is vulnerable to stones, which are created when there is an imbalance of cholesterol and bile salts, or when the bile duct fails to contract and empty its contents. Interestingly enough, excess estrogen can raise cholesterol levels and cause gallstones to form.

Liver cleansing herbs will accelerate the rate at which the liver gets rid of the toxins and xenoestrogens, preventing these harmful substances from doing further damage to the body, allowing the body to repair itself naturally and enabling herbal remedies to become more effective.

The liver cleanse also cleanses the gallbladder and helps to release stones held in the liver and gallbladder. The liver cleanse is also good for allergy relief, including clearing up skin problems such as rashes, hives and acne.

Do not start the liver cleanse until your bowels are moving 2-3 times a day, as your colon needs to be cleansed and fully functional for the liver cleanse to work effectively.

How To Do A Liver And Gallbladder Cleanse

The purpose of the liver cleanse is to release excess toxins from an overworked liver and to improve the overall functioning of the liver. It works by "fasting" your body for 12 hours so that your gallbladder can fill up with bile, then stimulating the gallbladder to release its bile contents to cleanse the liver and gallbladder. This has the effect of releasing stored toxins, fat, cholesterol and excess hormones.

The liver cleanse is best done in the morning, so that your fast is done overnight, and you prevent hunger pangs or low blood sugar issues from not eating for 12 hours. So if you have your evening meal at 7pm, you should be ready to start your cleanse at 7am in the morning without being hungry.

The liver cleanse involves taking a large amount of oil to stimulate the liver. You must take a "pure" oil, such as olive oil or flax seed oil, and for best results, use an organic, extra-virgin or cold-pressed oil.

The liver cleanse lasts for 5 days, and during the cleanse, you can eat a healthy diet making sure that you have a 12 hour fast before taking your oil and fruit juice. You can do a liver cleanse as many times as you like, as long as you take a week's break in between.

What To Do Each Day During Your 5-Day Liver Cleanse:

1. Drink a large glass of water immediately upon waking
2. Prepare and drink your liver flush drink
3. 20 minutes later take a Liver D-Tox Capsule
4. Drink a cup of Liver D-Tox Tea with breakfast
5. Take a Liver D-Tox Capsule and a cup of Liver D-Tox Tea with lunch and dinner

When you wake up, drink a large glass of water to clean out your digestive tract. After you've had your shower and are ready for breakfast, prepare your liver flush drink.

I've listed below the ingredients of the liver flush drink:

- 1 - 5 tablespoons of organic cold pressed oil such as olive oil or flax seed oil (On day 1, use one tablespoon, building up to 5 tablespoons by day 5.)
- 8oz (250ml) organic lemon or grapefruit, and orange juice (this should be freshly squeezed for best results)
- 8oz (250ml) filtered, distilled or spring or distilled water
- 1 inch of ginger

The easiest thing to do is put all the ingredients in the blender, hit the "on" switch and after a few seconds your drink will be ready. Using a blender makes the drink less oily tasting, and it's actually very filling.

Whatever you do, don't skip the ginger. Ginger makes the drink taste great, and most importantly, prevents you from feeling nausea if you are not used to oil.

If you love the taste of ginger, use an inch of a piece about as thick as your thumb. You can use less if you don't like the taste of ginger.

To make the liver cleanse even more potent, I suggest you add 1 to 5 cloves of garlic. This is probably one of the best healing foods around, and has several properties that will help you expel even more toxins.

You can eat normally during the day, but just remember to stop eating 12 hours before the next drink, as the liver flush drink should be taken on an empty stomach.

About 20 minutes after taking the liver flush drink, you will need to take a liver detox supplement. A liver detox supplement can contain one or more of the following herbs:

- Dandelion Root – helps to remove congestion from the liver by increasing the production of bile and flushing out excess fatty acids

- Garlic Bulb – a powerful disinfectant and natural antibiotic that kills viruses and harmful micro organisms, stimulates the immune system and repels parasites

- Ginger Root – combats nausea, reduces inflammation and kills viruses and bacteria

- Milk Thistle Seed –accelerates the growth of new liver cells, and protects the liver from being damaged by chemical toxins by strengthening the membranes of the liver cells

- Oregon Grape Root – stimulates the functioning of the liver and gallbladder, cleanses the blood and stimulates the production of bile

- Wormwood Leaf – kills parasites, reduces inflammation and supports the functioning of the liver

The Liver D-Tox Formula helps to stimulate liver detoxification. You will only need to take one capsule 3 times a day with meals for the duration of the 5-day liver cleanse.

You also need to drink a detox tea during the day, to help move the toxins out of your liver. The detox tea can contain any of the following herbs:

- Burdock Root – supports the liver in removing toxins and detoxifies the blood

- Cinnamon Bark – combats nausea, relieves intestinal gas and bloating and assists digestion

- Dandelion Root - helps to remove congestion from the liver by increasing the production of bile and flushing out excess fatty acids

- Fennel Seed – commonly used to break up stones and cleanse the liver and gallbladder

- Green Tea – lowers cholesterol, reduces inflammation and protects the liver from disease

- Licorice Root – stimulates the liver's production of bile, increases energy levels and balances estrogen levels

- Pau D'Arco Bark – reduces pain and inflammation, kills bacteria and micro organisms

- Peppermint Leaf – improves the flow of bile, helps the body break down gallstones and protects against viruses

The Liver D-Tox tea is easy to take. You can put a teaspoon into a cup and add boiling water then strain after letting it brew for 5 minutes, or put a tablespoon into a large jug and leave to cool, if you prefer to drink it cold. For best results, drink a few minutes before meals.

Taking the tea and capsules enable you to eat while doing the cleanse, while getting the same results as people who fast or follow a restrictive diet while cleansing.

Liver cleansing can increase your energy levels and help you maintain beautiful skin, clear eyes and a healthy metabolism.

Liver cleansing is vital if you want to balance your hormones to overcome conditions such as fibroids, endometriosis, PCOS, low sperm counts, low sex drives and even obesity.

Frequently Asked Questions

Question: Can I still do the liver cleanse if I have had my gallbladder removed?

Answer: Yes you can, but take the tea and capsules and not the liver flush drink.

Question: Can I add honey or sugar to the teas?

Answer: We do not recommend you add sweetenerg to the tea because sugar, honey and artificial sweeteners are not recommended as as part of a natural cleansing program.

If you are finding the teas too strong, leave them to steep for less time, dilute them with hot water, or add a small amount of stevia powder. (How much you add is entirely up to your own personal tastes. Stevia can be purchased at most health food stores, and is naturally sweet, but does not add calories, or affect blood sugar levels.

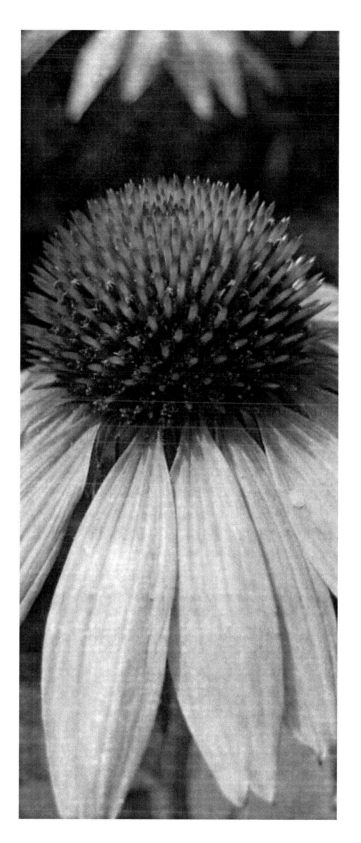

The kidneys and bladder are responsible for filtering waste products and cleansing the blood, and are one of your body's main detoxification and waste-disposal organs.

Cleansing the kidneys and bladder helps to strengthen the organs while removing built up waste that may clog the kidney's delicate filters.

Kidney And Bladder Cleansing

The kidneys are an important part of the urinary system, which consists of the kidneys, bladder, urethra and the tubes that connect the organs together. The kidneys are responsible for cleansing the blood, and getting rid of waste fluids via the urinary system.   They also regulate the blood pressure, volume of blood and the balance of salts and acids in the body.   The kidneys also secrete hormones that regulate bone formation and density.

The kidneys filter blood through a complex process of selecting essential nutrients for re-absorption by the body, removing waste materials and toxins from the blood, and managing the balance of fluids in the body. When the kidneys have done their job, the waste materials and excess fluids are transferred to the bladder for storage, where they are kept until the bladder is full and ready to release the waste via the urethra.

The kidneys filter approximately 180 liters of blood, and are easily overloaded with toxins as our modern lifestyles require us to consume foods that the body was not designed to handle.   For example, commercial foods sprayed with pesticides, and pumped full of additives and preservatives will require your kidneys to filter our the chemicals to clean the blood.

Even having a sluggish colon filled with intestinal waste can cause toxins and waste to be reabsorbed into the blood stream, putting extra strain on the kidneys.   Fatty and high carbohydrate foods also thicken the blood, with increased fat and glucose molecules that require filtering by the kidneys.

When the kidneys are overloaded, some of the materials that should be filtered out remain inside the kidneys, causing irritation and inflammation. Sometimes the materials can crystallize and form stones, which can either get stuck and grow larger, or pass through the kidney can urinary system, damaging the tissues and causing considerable pain to the person with the kidney stone.

The combination of thick, over-toxic blood, and the kidney's reduced ability to filter it require the heart to increase the pressure of blood flow to enable the thickened blood to move through the kidney's filters. This results in high blood pressure, which causes further damage to the kidneys.

The bladder is also prone to infection – especially in women. Bladder infections can be caused by excess sugar in the urine, sexual activity, antibiotics, commercial soaps and douches and spermicides. Bladder infections, and infections of the urinary tract can be extremely painful, and harmful to the kidneys if left untreated.

You can often detect someone's state of health by the quality and quantity of their urine. Someone in good health should urinate around 4 to 6 times a day, and expel 1 to 2 quarts a day (this is roughly 1 to 2 liters). Healthy urine should be transparent, but slightly tinted in color, and have no odor. Many people have dark colored, strong smelling urine, which is an indication of poor health or poor lifestyle.

What To Do Each Day During Your 5-Day Kidney Cleanse:

1. **Drink a large glass of water immediately upon waking**
2. **Prepare and drink your kidney flush drink**
3. **20 minutes later take a Kidney D-Tox Capsule**
4. **Drink a cup of Kidney D-Tox Tea with breakfast**
5. **Take a Liver D-Tox Capsule and a cup of Liver D-Tox Tea with lunch and dinner**

How To Do A Kidney Cleanse

Drink a large glass of water when you wake up, to flush out the digestive and urinary tract.

Next, prepare a kidney flush drink. This formula is based on Stanley Burrough's Master Cleanse drink, which contains the following ingredients:

- 1 lemon or lime, juiced

- 16oz (half a liter) of water

- A pinch of Cayenne Pepper

The best way to prepare this is to put all the ingredients into a blender and mix for 15 seconds.

About 20 minutes after drinking the kidney cleansing drink, take a Kidney D-Tox Capsule. It contains:

- Burdock Root – purifies the blood to toxins, increases the flow of urine and neutralizes acidic urine

- Corn Silk – increases the flow of urine and reduces pain and inflammation in the urinary tract

- Gravel Root – breaks down kidney stones, reduces inflammation in the bladder and urethra, and helps the body fight cystitis and pelvic inflammatory disease

- Horsetail Herb – strengthens inflamed and over stressed kidneys, and increases the flow of urine

- Hydrangea Root – a natural diuretic that increases the flow of urine, and strengthens the mucus membranes of the urinary tract

- Juniper Berries – natural antibacterial and anti fungal properties, reduces inflammation and water retention and increases the flow of urine

- Marshmallow Root – coats the tissues of the urinary tract to soothe inflammation and eases the passage of stones, contains compounds that neutralize toxins , used to treat interstitial cystitis

- Uva Ursi Leaves – strengthens the lining of the urinary tract, and kills bacteria that causes bladder infection

The Kidney D-Tox formula helps cleanse the kidneys and bladder by purifying the blood, putting less strain on the kidneys, increasing the flow of urine through the urinary tract without raising blood pressure, and reducing inflammation and infection, allowing the kidney's filters to work more efficiently. This formula can be taken 3 times a day with meals.

To make your kidney cleanse even more effective prepare a tea containing at least one of the following herbs:

- Alfalfa Herb – reduces inflammation and neutralizes acids, and is rich in nutrients that strengthen the kidneys and bladder

- Echinacea – reduces tissue damage and edema in the kidney, enhances the immune system to fight infection, and speeds up healing

- Goldenseal – powerful natural antibiotic and antiseptic, especially when combined with Echinacea, reduces inflammation and helps the body fight infection

- Licorice Root – strengthens the kidneys, heals damaged tissues, purifies the blood and reduces cholesterol

- Nettle Leaf – helps the body maintain a healthy electrolyte balance, reduces inflammation and assists detoxification of the blood

- Parsley Root – manages water levels, dissolves stones, and clears uric acid from the urinary tract

- Rosemary Leaf – reduces inflammation, kills bacteria, reduces kidney pains and relieves pain and spasms in the bladder

- Wild Yam – reduces spasms in the bladder an urinary tract, treats nausea and reduces inflammation

The Kidney D-Tox tea is easy to take. You can put a teaspoon into a cup and add boiling water then strain after letting it brew for 5 minutes, or put a tablespoon into a large jug and leave to cool, if you prefer to drink it cold. For best results, drink a few minutes before meals.

You can eat your meals as normal while doing the kidney cleanse, but be careful to increase your intake of fresh water, to enhance the benefits of the cleanse.

To maintain healthy kidneys, cut out coffee, black teas and sodas, and drink water, fruit and vegetable juices, and herbal teas instead.

You can also support your kidneys by taking vitamin A and E supplements, eating parsley, green peas and dark green vegetables.

Frequently Asked Questions

Question: I am urinating more often than usual. Is that normal?

Answer: Yes many of the herbs in the Kidney Cleansing Program have diuretic qualities, so increased urination is completely normal. Ensure that you're drinking plenty of water to flush out your system every day. 8 glasses of fluid a day is ideal (this includes the consumed in your teas.)

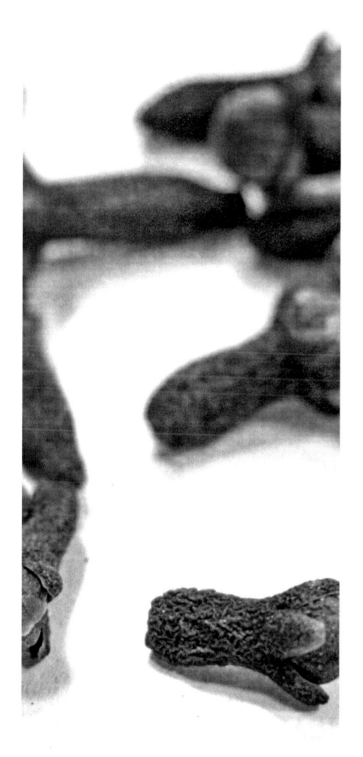

Parasites and heavy metals are responsible for a range of symptoms that are easily misdiagnosed, and completing a 5-day Toxin Cleanse can help increase the effectiveness of your cleanses, and get rid of any unexplained symptoms you may have as a result of parasites or heavy metals.

Toxin Cleansing

After completing the three major body cleanses, you will begin to feel lighter, healthier and stronger. Many people have reported shedding excess weight, improved energy levels and even fertility boosts simply after following the first three cleanses!

To make your cleanses even more powerful, and to get the full benefits from herbal remedies, diets or health programs, you would do well to consider toxin cleansing. This is the final stage of a body cleanse program, and includes:

- Parasite cleansing

- Heavy metal cleansing

Parasite Cleanse

Parasites are everywhere; you can pick them up from contaminated water, restaurant food, undercooked meat and dairy products, unwashed fruits and vegetables, your pets, overseas travel and even other people.   One medical doctor reported that approximately 80% of his patients had suffered a parasitic infection at one point in their lives.

The most common type of parasite are intestinal parasites. Some nest in the small intestines, where they can feed on the nutrients in your food, preventing you from absorbing the nutrients you need.   Others stay in the large intestine, and cause symptoms that mimic irritable bowel syndrome and other digestive disorders.

It is important to rid yourself of parasites because they cause a range of diseases, and symptoms including digestive upsets, skin complaints, depression, fatigue, low blood sugar, obesity, sleeping problems and allergies. Parasites can stay in the body undetected for years, as their symptoms often mimic common diseases such as colitis, ulcers and diabetes.

They also over-stimulate the immune system, leaving you vulnerable to colds and infections, which put your body in a weakened state. Medical researchers have linked problems in the immune system with unexplained infertility and recurrent miscarriage. Researchers in the USA have found that reducing the immune response in a group of women who had failed to conceive helped nearly 80% them to become pregnant.

The most effective way to get rid of these parasites is via herbal remedies. While medication can get rid of one or two different species of parasite, there are take three herbs to kill over a hundred different species of parasite without side effects.

The most common anti-parasitical herbs are:

- Black Walnut – kills intestinal parasites, worms, fungus and yeast, cleanses the blood and aids digestion and stimulates the flow of fecal matter

- Cloves – kills parasite eggs, reduce nausea, inflammation and infection

- Wormwood – kills and expels worms from the organs and intestinal system, and strengthens the liver, gallbladder and digestive system

Para D-Tox is a complete herbal solution for killing parasites, and contains ingredients that kill and expel over 100 known parasites.

If you are doing the Parasite Cleanse as part of the Total Body Cleansing Program (or you purchased a Body Cleanse Kit), 5 days will be enough to get you results, as the colon and liver cleanses will have already killed a lot of parasites.

If you are doing the parasite cleanse as a stand-alone parasite detoxification program, you will need to take Para D-Tox 3 times a day for a month, but do a colon cleanse first, in order to clear a path for the intestinal parasites to exit the body.

Eating raw garlic, oregano and raw onions help kill parasites. They can be easily incorporated into salads and salad dressings, or added to sandwiches or wraps to give you extra protection against parasitic pests.

Heavy Metal Cleanse

Heavy metal toxicity can have a huge negative impact on your health, hormones and fertility, and can affect virtually every organ in your body.

Three common toxic metals are lead, aluminum and mercury. People tend to pick up of heavy metal poisoning from drinking water, contaminated fish, lead pipes, cigarette smoke, mercury amalgam tooth fillings, cooking utensils and deodorant.

If you have more than two fillings in your teeth and would like to give yourself the best chance of conceiving, you should consider removing the mercury fillings from your teeth, and replacing them with non- toxic materials such as porcelain. If you decide to remove the mercury in your mouth, you need to visit a dentist who specializes in removing mercury amalgam fillings.

Fish is another common source of heavy metal toxicity. The US Environmental Protection Agency states:

"Nearly all fish and shellfish contain traces of mercury. For most people, the risk from mercury by eating fish and shellfish is not a health concern. Yet, some fish and shellfish contain higher levels of mercury that may harm an unborn baby or young child's developing nervous system. The risks from mercury in fish and shellfish depend on the amount of fish and shellfish eaten and the levels of mercury in the fish and shellfish. Therefore, the Food and Drug Administration (FDA) and the Environmental Protection Agency (EPA) are advising women who may become pregnant, pregnant women, nursing mothers, and young children to avoid some types of fish and eat fish and shellfish that are lower in mercury."

Heavy metals, especially lead, have also been identified to cause infertility. In a Germany hospital, researchers found that women with high levels of heavy metal in their blood were most likely to suffer from hormone disorders, uterine fibroids and miscarriages. When they chelated the heavy metals from a group of infertile women, they found that many of them became pregnant without medical assistance.

Two important herbs for removing metal from the body are cilantro (coriander) and chlorella. Cilantro (coriander) can help your body to chelate (cleanse) mercury through your urine. For faster results, you can take chlorella. These herbs are a cost-effective and gentle alternative to EDTA therapy.

- Cilantro – neutralizes heavy metals, allowing them to be released from the body's tissues

- Chlorella – absorbs heavy metals from the blood stream and tissues, allowing them to be safely removed by the urinary system

Metal D-Tox can help you remove heavy metals without side effects, as its ingredients bind themselves to the heavy metals, so they can be safely removed by the liver and urinary system.

If you are doing the Metal Cleanse as part of the Body Cleansing Program (or have purchased a Body Cleanse Kit), take Metal D-Tox 3 times a day for 5 days with meals.

As a "stand alone" Metal Cleansing Program, you will need to take a capsule of Metal D-Tox 3 times a day with meals for at least 3 weeks.

Frequently Asked Questions

Question: I got pregnant after doing the Kidney Cleanse - should I take Para D-Tox and Metal D-Tox

 now?

Answer: Stop cleansing as soon as you get pregnant, and switch to AlkaGreens Plus, which contains ingredients that provide a mild and even safer detoxification effect.

Question: Do I take Para D-Tox at the same time as Metal D-Tox?

Answer: Yes, you can take them both at the same time.

Question: I'm confused - how long to I need to do the toxin cleanse for?

Answer: If you have purchased the Body Cleanse Kit, do the toxin cleanse for 5 days, as the previous cleanses will have already removed a lot of toxins from your body, so 5 days will be enough to get good results.

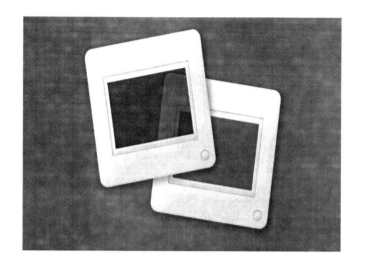

Herbal remedies are effective for helping the body shed its stores of excess fat, increasing the metabolic rate, and reducing your cravings for specific foods. Recent research has indicated that specific herbs can block the body's absorption of fats and calories, making them ideal for speeding up weight loss.

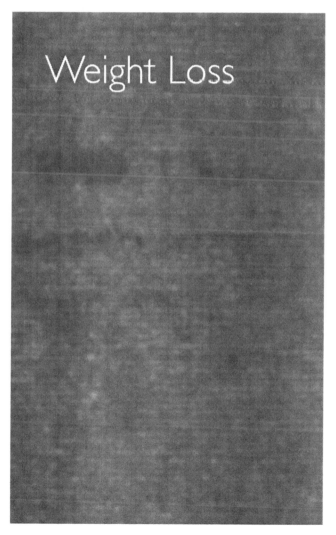

Weight Loss

Remedies For Weight Loss

Approximately one-third of Americans are overweight or obese, and the figures for other industrialized countries are catching up with the USA.

Contrary to popular belief, obesity is not a disorder associated with those with a lack of willpower, neglect, or poor dietary choices. It can affect anybody, regardless of background, exercise levels or diet.

Obesity results from a complex interaction of many factors, such as metabolism, hormonal imbalance, endocrine diseases, and blood sugar fluctuations, so treating obesity isn't as simple as "eating less and exercising more".

Obesity has been cited as the number one contributing factor to diseases such as diabetes, heart disease, autoimmune diseases such as arthritis, and even some cancers. In addition, specialists suggest that losing even five to ten percent of your body weight can be beneficial in preventing these diseases.

Being overweight, and more specifically, having a Body Mass Index over over 25 can affect your fertility, and researchers have linked being overweight to developing Polycystic Ovarian Syndrome (PCOS) in women. This condition can make mentruation more irregular and disrupt ovulation, reducing your chances of conceiving. Similarly, in men, being overweight can also increase the fat around the testes, and provide an unwanted layer of insulation, which can raise the temperature (and lower the vitality) of sperm.

The good news is that you don't have to reach your goal weight to conceive. Just reducing your weight by 5-10% of your current weight is enough to significantly improve your fertility. The key to improving your fertility by changing your diet is to lower the insulin levels by cutting down on refined carbohydrates and eating good quality organic sources of meat and vegetable proteins, combined with organic fruits and vegetables.

Why Most Diets Do Not Work

95% of all documented cases of diets have failed for the following reasons:

- Fad diets that completely restrict a food group are unrealistic in the long run, these diets focus mainly on weight loss for cosmetic reasons. Your body needs a well balanced diet, and that includes some carbohydrates to function properly.

- Research has shown that as soon as the dieter reaches their goal, they go right back to the unhealthy way of eating and gain all the weight back.

- It is unreasonable to weigh and measure everything you eat, and many people who eat out, or eat at work or school are unable to stick to strict diets because of this.

- Diets lower your metabolism, as the body recognizes a shortage of food, and slows down the rate at which it converts calories into energy. The next time you eat your body stores most of the food eaten as fat because it anticipates the starvation.

For these reasons nutritionists, herbalists and naturopaths suggest using herbal remedies to deter hunger, block fat absorption, and boost metabolism.

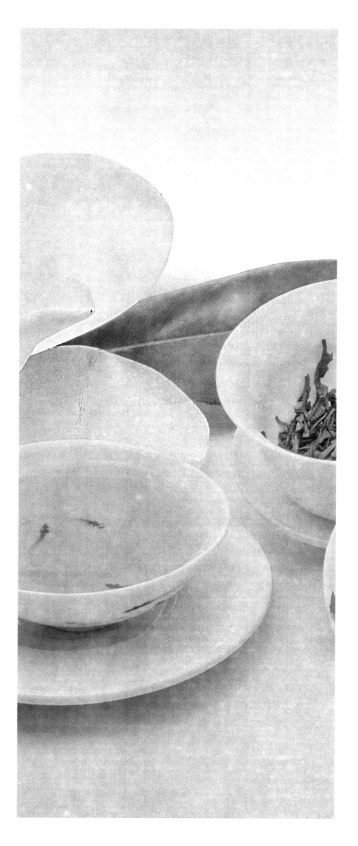

Wulong-Oolong is a rare species of oolong tea, grown in a small plantation in the Wuyi Mountains of Fujian, China – the location of some of the finest and rarest teas in the world. It is currently used in $1,500-a day Hollywood health spas to help their clients burn maximum fat.

Wulong-Oolong

Wulong Oolong can help you accelerate your weight loss because:

Oolong tea increases your fat burning ability by 12%. Scientists at the University of Tokushima found that men consuming a "typical American diet" increased their rate of fat burning by 12% and boosted calories burned 3.4% when drinking Oolong tea.

Oolong tea is 250% more effective for boosting the metabolism than Green Tea. Researchers from The Tokushima School of Medicine discovered that Oolong tea increased energy expenditure by 10%, compared to the 4% increase from green tea, making Oolong tea 250% more effective at boosting the metabolism than green tea.

The polyphenols in Oolong tea block the absorption of dietary fat and cholesterol by over 50%. Researchers at the The University of Tokushima discovered that subjects on a high fat diet drinking Oolong tea 3 times a day with meals absorbed half the amount of dietary fat and cholesterol than those who did not drink the tea.

Oolong tea prevents obesity, even while eating a high-fat diet. Researchers at Ehime School of Medicine reduced the body's absorption of lipids, and increased the rate fats were burned by giving subjects Oolong tea.

Oolong tea helps to reduce abdominal fat safely. Researchers at the Teikyo University School of Medicine discovered that the catechins in oolong tea helped to reduce abdominal fat without influencing the absorption of fat-soluble vitamins.

Oolong tea reduces LDL cholesterol. In a randomized controlled clinical trial, researchers at Osaka City University Medical School gave 22 patients with coronary artery disease 1 liter of Oolong tea for a month, and discovered a significant reduction in plasma adiponectin levels, and a reduction in plasma level LDL particle size, and a significant difference in hemoglobin A1c levels after drinking Oolong tea.

Oolong tea prevents hypertension. In a study of 1507 people, doctors at the, National Cheng Kung University Medical did a study found that people who drank tea on a daily basis were significantly less likely to develop hypertension.

Oolong tea helps to reduce stress. Researchers at the Academy of Traditional Chinese Medicine of Fujian Province found that taking 4 servings of Oolong tea a day for a week reduced stress levels significantly, decreased cortisol levels (the stress hormone) and increased mental alertness.

The fragrant aroma of Oolong tea stimulates relaxation. Researchers at Yamaguchi University found that the fragrant compounds in oolong tea stimulated the GABA receptors of the brain. These are the parts of the brain that releases a chemical that reduces muscle.

Ingredients
100% Wuyi Oolong tea

Also available in capsule form.

How To Make A Cup Of Tea
Place a teaspoon of Wulong-Oolong into a cup, and add water. Leave to seep for 3-5 minutes, then strain and serve.

If you prefer your tea to be sweet, add half a teaspoon of stevia powder to it.

Wulong Oolong can also be made into iced tea, and kept refrigerated for 48 hours.

Drink a cup of Wulong-Oolong with every meal for best results.

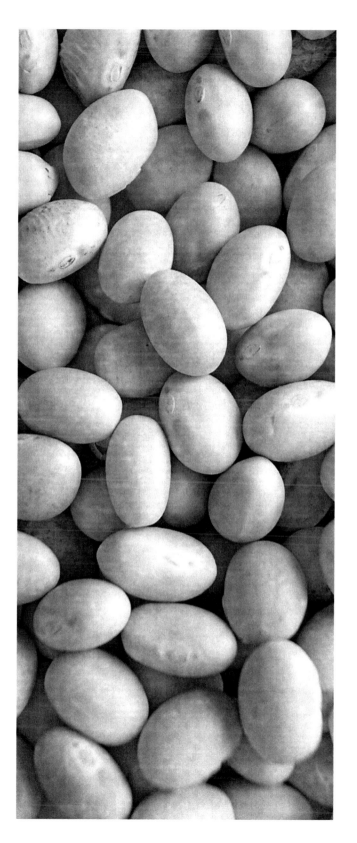

CarboClear contains natural ingredients that prevent carbohydrates and sugars from being broken down and absorbed by the body, and ingredients that help the body expel the undigested carbohydrates.

CarboClear

Carboclear is designed to:

- Block carbohydrate absorption by disrupting the conversion of complex carbohydrates into absorbable sugars

- Make dieting more efficient - a study at the University of California resulted in subjects losing an average of 8.7 pounds and 3.3 inches from their waists

- Reduce the accumulation of fatty acids in the liver, and is scientifically proven to prevent obesity

- Assist the body in disposing of excess glucose can carbohydrates, without storing it as body fat

- Accelerate fat loss, and helps to maintain lean muscle mass while following a reduced calorie diet

- Balance blood sugar and reduce food cravings

- Reduce hunger by 37%, and suppress the appetite

- Increase energy levels and help the body to cope with stress, preventing comfort eating

Ingredients

White Kidney Bean Extract

White kidney beans reduce the absorption of calories from carbohydrates by disrupting alpha-amylase – the digestive enzyme responsible for converting carbohydrates into simple absorbable sugars. It has been scientifically proven to block carbohydrate absorption and in a clinical study at the University of California, subjects lost on average 8.7 pounds and 3.3 inches from their waists while taking white kidney bean extract.

Doctors from the UCLA School of Medicine recently published reports that white kidney bean extract tripled the amount of weight lost by dieters taking the supplement. In addition, scientists from Rome, Italy concluded that white kidney bean extract reduced fat mass and helped maintain lean muscle mass even in dieters who had struggled to lose weight for 6 months.

Fenugreek Seed

Fenugreek is a commonly used culinary herb, which has a number of health benefits for dieters. Researchers at Tokyo University found that fenugreek seed prevented obesity in subjects following a high calorie diet, and scientists at the University of Waterloo, Canada confirmed that the herb reduced the accumulation of fat in the liver.

Fenugreek is rich in 4-hydroxyisoleucine, an amino acid that controls blood sugar.. According to recent findings at the University of Yaounde, taking fenugreek with meals reduces food intake in future meals, as the herb reduces the transit times of carbohydrates, which has an effect of balancing blood sugar and reducing food cravings.

Cinnamon Bark

Cinnamon is a culinary spice used for flavoring foods, and has several medical benefits for dieters. Cinnamon contains dihydroxyhydrocinnamic acid, a naturally-occurring plant extract that helps the body dispose of glucose and carbohydrates, without storing it as body fat. Swedish researchers at Malmo University identified cinnamon as a natural appetite suppressant, which slowed hunger by 37%, when taken with meals.

Its active component cinnamaldehyde is currently under research as a anti-diabetic treatment, due to its blood glucose balancing effects. Researchers have found that when cinnamon is combined with other herbs, it can lower blood glucose levels and help increase insulin sensitivity, which proves promising for curing insulin resistance and metabolic syndrome.

American Ginseng

American ginseng has been used in Native American medicine to increase energy levels, balance blood sugar levels and help the mind and body deal with stress – a common cause of over eating. American ginseng also prevents energy slumps throughout the day, which is another common cause of over eating.

Its fat burning benefits were confirmed by reports from University of Chicago, which recommended American ginseng for weight loss and the prevention of diabetes. Researchers at the Kyung Hee University, Korea also found that the herb prevented obesity.

How To Take CarboClear

Take 3-4 capsules of CarboClear with a high carbohydrate meal or snack.

Frequently Asked Questions

Question: How does CarboClear work?

Amswer: Its ingredients act as amylase inhibitors, which stop the enzyme responsible for breaking down carbohydrates and allowing them to pass through the small intestine into the bloodstream, where they raise insulin levels and are converted into fat.

Instead, the carbohydrates move undigested into the large intestine, where they are turned into feces.

Question: Should I take CarboClear every day?

Answer: Although its ingredients are safe to be taken every day, CarboClear was designed as a way for you to enjoy the occasional high carbohydrate meal or snack without gaining weight.

Question: Does CarboClear block fats?

Answer: No, CarboClear only blocks the absorption of carbohydrates. For an effective fat blocker, use LipoClear:

Success Story

"I am in a wheelchair and don't have many options for exercising so tried Wulong-Oolong, CarboClear and LipoClear to see if it would help me lose weight.

I did not need to add any sweeteners to it, as it was very pleasant tasting. The capsules didn't taste of anything, and were easy enough to swallow.

In my first week I lost 3.5 pounds then 2 pounds the second week, and since then I've been avearaging 1 to 1.5 pounds a week."

Marie Crean, Waterford, Ireland

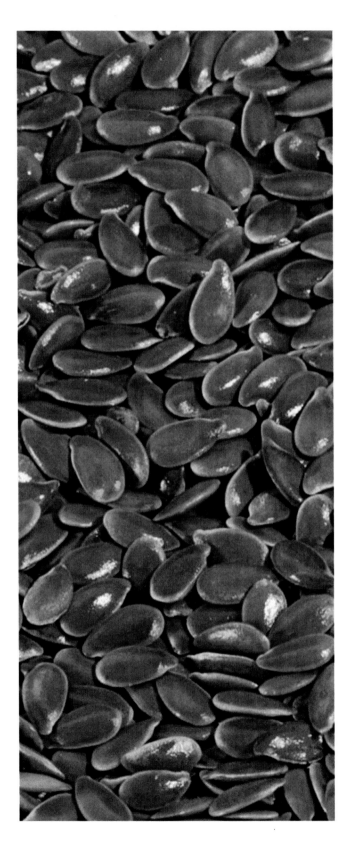

LipoClear is a natural fat-blocker supplement that prevents the absorption of dietary fats, and helps the body to dispose of dietary fat without storing it as body fat.

LipoClear

LipoClear contains ingredients that prevent the fats you eat from being deposited into your fat cells, and can:

- Prevent fats from being digested, and assists the body in getting rid of dietary fat without storing it as body fat

- Increase the feelings of "fullness" and satisfaction with meals by 27.1%, and scientifically proven to result in eating 15.8% less food in subsequent meals

- Lower the glycemic index of meals

- Increase the metabolism of fats and can help dieters lose an average of 13 pounds without hunger of cravings

- Prevent stress-related weight gain by preventing the release of hormones that cause fat to accumulate around the middle

- Contain thermogenic ingredients that raise the metabolism safely

- Control the expansion of fat cells

Ingredients

Psyllium Husks

Psyllium comes from the seeds of the Plantago Ovata plant, and are a natural source of soluble fiber. The Pennington Biomedical Research Center found that consuming psyllium husks with high fat diets can prevent weight gain, and researchers at Kings College University of London found that subjects felt fuller after taking psyllium hulls, and as a result, ate less fat in subsequent meals.

According to findings at Massey University, New Zealand, the soluble dietary fibers from psyllium and guar gum alter the digestion of fats. Taking psyllium with foods high in fat prevents the fats from being digested and absorbed by the body. Researchers at the Oasis of Hope Hospital in Mexico confirmed that the fat leaves the body in feces, and these findings were confirmed by the University of Wisconsin-Green Bay, who concluded that dietary fats became less digestible with psyllium.

Guar gum

Guar gum comes from guar beans, and is a highly soluble fiber that attaches itself to fat particles in food, preventing the body's absorption of dietary fats. Scientists at the University of Agriculture in Pakistan found that guar gum helped to lower the glycemic index of meals – when consumed with guar gum, and helped lower blood glucose and cholesterol levels, assisting weight loss.

Guar gum is a natural appetite suppressant, as it is bulk forming, and increases satisfaction with meals. Researchers at Abbott Laboratories found that the fiber in guar gum resulted in a 27.1% increase in fullness after meals, and a 15.8% decrease in food consumption.

Green Tea

Green tea is recognized word-wide as a beneficial health drink, and has been used for thousands of years in China to help manage weight. This has been confirmed by recent clinical trials at the Universitary Medicine Berlin, where doctors reported that the epigallocatechin-3-gallate substances in green tea increased the rate of fat burning in overweight patients.

Scientists at Maastricht University, Netherlands found that the catechins in green tea prevent stress-related weight gain by suppressing the enzyme catechol o-methyltransferase, which triggers the release of stress-hormones that cause fat to accumulate in the abdomen. Another clinical study at Maastricht University resulted in 76 men and women losing an average of 13 pounds (5.9 kgs) without hunger or cravings.

Cayenne (90,000 H.U.)

Cayenne is a hot chilli pepper used in Chinese and South American cooking, and has been used in Native American medicine for at least 9,000 years. It's active component, capsaicin is a naturally thermogenic food, as it raises the body's production of heat, increasing metabolism and fat burning.

Clinical trials at the University of Tasmania, Australia found that chili lowered the body's insulin production after high calorie meals, meaning less nutrients are absorbed as fat. When combined with green tea, capsaicin has a significant effect on controlling the expansion of fat cells.

How To Take LipoClear

Take 3-4 capsules of LipoClear with high fat meals or snacks.

Do not take LipoClear with omega oil, flaxseed oil, or fish oil supplements, as LipoClear will prevent the body from using these beneficial fats.

Frequently Asked Questions

Question: Why should I take LipoClear separately from oil-based supplements?

Answer: LipoClear is a powerful fat blocker and does not discriminate against the quality of the fat it blocks. This means it is capable of blocking fat-soluble vitamins, omega oils and fish oil supplements.

Question: I take omega oil supplements but I want to lose weight with LipoClear. What should I do?

Answer: We recommend you take your fat supplements 2 hours before or after taking LipoClear.

Question: Should I take LipoClear every day?

Answer: LipoClear was designed to be taken as a way to prevent weight gain from the occasional fatty meal, and is not a replacement for a sensible diet and exercise program.

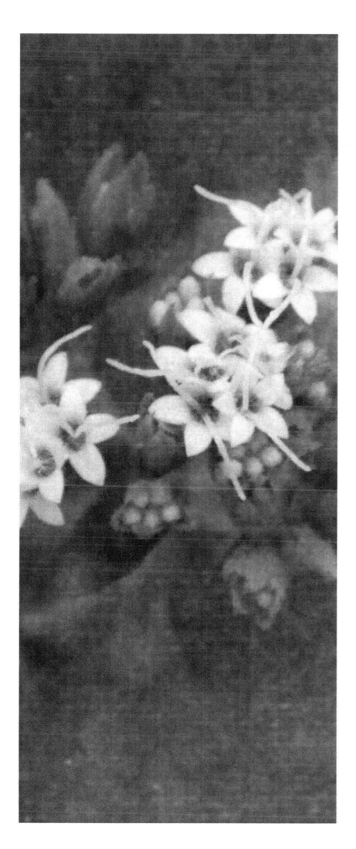

CraveEx is designed to help you curb your cravings for carbohydrates and sweet foods, while supporting your efforts in losing weight. CraveEx can be taken every day with meals, to help you beat the habit of eating unhealthy foods.

CraveEx

CraveEx is particularly useful if you have problems sticking to your diet due to constant food cravings, hunger, or energy slumps. It contains ingredients that help you feel more satisfied with your meals, and can:

- Reduce the cravings for carbohydrates and sweet foods

- Make sugary foods taste less sweet, and reduce your desire to overeat

- Prevent hypoglycemia and manages blood sugar levels, preventing overeating

- Stimulate weight loss and increases the metabolic rate

- Optimize the metabolism of carbohydrates

- Slow down the development no fat cells, and reduces abdominal fat

- Help detoxify the liver and digestive system

Ingredients

Gymnema Leaf

Gymnema leaf has been used for thousands of years in Ayurvedic medicine to prevent obesity, balance blood sugar levels. Gymnema leaf is particularly beneficial for people craving carbohydrates and sweet foods, as research from Kyushu University, Japan confirms that the herb can make sugary foods taste less sweet, and reduce the desire to eat more.

Human studies at the Georgetown University Medical Center have confirmed that gymnema is a safe, non-toxic and effective weight loss herb that helps reduce excess body fat and Body Mass Index.

Stevia Extract 85% Stevioside

Stevia leaves have been used for hundreds of years in Paraguy and Brazil as a natural sweetener. Although stevia is naturally 300 times sweeter than sugar, it contains no calories, and has been scientifically proven by the University of Maringa, Brazil, to prevent hypoglycemia – a common cause of sugar cravings, and balance blood sugar levels naturally.

Stevia's active ingredient, stevioside has been commended by the Catholic University of Leuven, Belgium, to be a non-toxic, supplement for preventing overeating and stimulating weight loss.

Licorice Root

Licorice root is a sweet herb that is naturally low in calories. It is a popular sweetener for medicines, soft drinks and candies, and in its natural root form, can curb cravings for sweet or carbohydrate-rich foods. Licorice is a common ingredient for detoxification and digestion remedies, as it has beneficial effects for liver health and fuction.

Japanese researchers found that the flavionids in licorice prevent the liver from converting nutrients into fat, and further research indicates that licorice is effective in increasing the metabolic rate, optimizing the metabolism of carbohydrates and lowering abdominal fat. The National Institute of Child Health and Human Development have linked licorice extract to slowing down the development of fat cells.

Dandelion Root

Dandelion balances blood sugar levels – the University of Bologna, Italy identified the herb as a natural treatment for hypoglycemia. Koren researchers at Yeungnam University found that dandelion extract improved the metabolism of fats and reduced sugar imbalances in human subjects.

Dandelion root is a powerful detoxification herb, especially when combined with licorice root. European herbalists have used dandelion for hundreds of years to strengthen the digestive system and liver. It is also a rich source of Vitamin A, B complex, Vitamins C, D, calcium, potassium and zinc.

How To Take CraveEx

Take one capsule with meals, 3 times a day to help reduce cravings.

Frequently Asked Questions

Question: Is it okay for me to take CraveEx every day?

Answer: Yes! CraveEx was designed to be taken every day to help you reduce food cravings and prevent you from eating between meals due to hunger pangs or energy slumps.

Question: Is CraveEx an appetite suppressant?

Answer: While some of the ingredients can reduce overeating, it works by balancing the blood sugar levels, which has a secondary effect of keeping energy levels high, and making you less likely to eat between meals.

CraveEx can stop overeating, but will not prevent you from enjoying 3 balanced meals a day.

Question: I'm confused. Which of the weight loss supplements should I take if I want to lose weight?

Answer: It all depends on what you want to acheive. If you are looking for a way to increase your metabolism, we recommend you drink Wulong-Oolong with every meal.

If you plan on enjoying the occasional high carbohydrate and high fat meal, but do not want to gain weight, then we recommend you take CarboClear and LipoClear with these types of meals.

If your problem is overeating, food cravings, or feeling a lack of energy when you're dieting, and you would like to stick to your diet and increase your energy levels without adding calories, we recommend CraveEx.

People who have had excellent results in losing large amounts of weight have followed a complete program consisting of:

- A 4-week body cleanse- with the Body Cleanse Kit
- Taking AlkaGreens Plus with vegetable juice each morning before exercise
- Drinking Wulong-Oolong with every meal
- Taking CarboClear 3 times a day to reduce cravings
- Following a balanced diet with plenty of organic fresh fruit and vegetables, vegetarian and fish proteins, and complex carbohydrates and whole grains
- Drinking 8 glasses of water each day
- 3 "Cheat meals" a week, with LipoClear and CarboClear

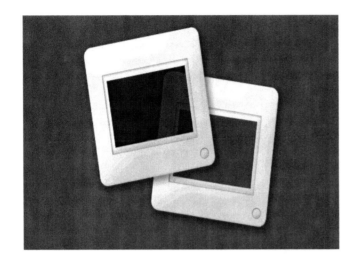

If you have been struggling to conceive for 12 months or more, consider combining a herbal cleansing program with herbal remedies, natural fertility techniques such as yoga and massage, with a food-based supplement such as AlkaGreens Plus.

Fertility

Remedies For Fertility

It's common knowledge amongst medical professionals that most fertility problems are caused by hormonal imbalances. For example, an excess of estrogen can cause conditions such as fibroids and endometriosis, which cause fertility challenges.

And imbalances in Follicle Stimulating Hormone and Luteinizing Hormone can also reduce or stop menstruation, and make ovulation infrequent, giving you less chances to conceive.

Similarly, men with low sperm counts often lack sufficient levels of testosterone to produce the millions of healthy motile sperm required to conceive a baby.

Toxicity is also a common cause of unexplained infertility, as well as the rise in reproductive complaints such as low sex drive, endometriosis, fibroids, PCOS, low sperm counts, and blocked fallopian tubes.

Is Infertility A Female Problem?

Statistics indicate that 40% of infertility is due to male factor infertility, with low sperm counts being the primary causes.

Unfortunately, an increasing number of men are being diagnosed with low sperm counts, poor motility and high rates of abnormally formed sperm cells.

For example, in the UK, the average sperm count has fallen from 110 million per ml of semen to 70 million per ml. Figures for the rest of Europe, USA, Australia and New Zealand are also following this trend.

In fact, figures from the World Health Organization suggest the average sperm count has fallen 50% world-wide in the past 50 years.

So what is making the difference? Studies indicate that lifestyle factors are largely to blame for the declining sperm counts and sperm quality. Both men and women are exposed to toxic fumes, pesticides in fruits and vegetables and fertility-damaging chemicals in household products.

Similarly, cigarettes, alcohol, poor diets and nutritionally deficient foods contribute to the lower sperm counts and other sperm-related

problems such as poor motility, vitality a morphology. A significant amount of nutrition is needed to create sperm, and the average Western diet does not provide many men with the nutrients they need to stay healthy, let alone reproduce.

Environmental toxins, chemicals in food, water and cosmetics are not the only cause. Free radicals also damage DNA and can result in a high percentage of deformed and dead or dying sperm.

In fact, doctors have found that men with sperm vitality problems have higher concentrations of free radicals in their semen than men with normal, healthy sperm.

Advice For Both Men And Women

Combining herbal remedies with a toxin-cleansing program, such as the Body Cleanse Kit can significantly increase your chances of conceiving, especially when combined with a healthy, balanced, nutrient-rich diet.

Antioxidants can help improve the quality of sperm and eggs, and lead to less miscarriages, birth defects and a healthier pregnancy. Consider taking AntioxiPlus alongside your FertilPlus supplements.

Additionally, AlkaGreens Plus can provide you with the equivalent of a day's servings of superfood fruit and vegetables in just one scoop.

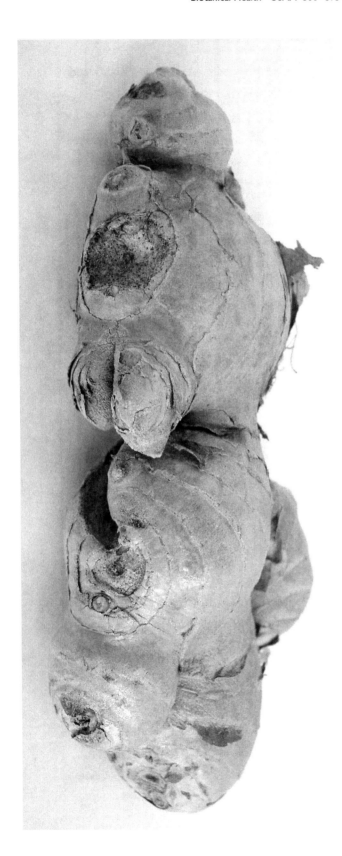

FertilPlus For Men is a herbal supplement to help increase male sperm count, sperm motility and sperm vitality.

FertilPlus For Men

FertilPlus For Men is designed to help increase male fertility over a period of 90 days - the time it takes to produce new sperm. It also provides the following fertility-boosting benefits:

- Increase sperm count by 31% and increase semen volume by 34%

- Double sperm count, while increasing sperm survival rate

- Increase free testosterone levels, and provide the body with plant steroids for transformation into testosterone

- Improve sex drive and improve sexual function in men

- Protect the male reproductive system against environmental stress and chemical pollution

- Maintain the health of the male reproductive and urinary tract, and protect the prostate gland

- Boost the energy levels, and help the body cope with mental and physical stress

You Helped Save Our Marriage
And My Wife's Now Pregnant!

Sorry for the long letter but words cannot succinctly express how much the support and advice you've generously shared with me have changed my life.

I'm 52 and my wife is 43.

The constant strain of conceiving caused many arguments between us. We only made love when she was ovulating, and I felt I couldn't give her the emotional support she needed.

I was also very sensitive whenever she brought up the "baby issue" as I knew I was the sole cause of our failure to conceive.

One day, I arrived home from work and found she'd gone. She left a note saying she couldn't stay married to someone who didn't care about having a baby, and she'd gone to her sister's to think about things.

That was a real wake-up call for me. Whilst I cared as much as she did, I wasn't showing that I cared, and had also resigned myself to being infertile. Thankfully someone recommended your services and I followed your program to the letter.

Here are the results I achieved after following your programme:

	1 Mar 2006	1 Jun 2006	1 Sep 2006
Volume	1.8ml	2.9ml	3.8ml
Ph	7.1	7.4	7.4
Count	11.9 million/ml	18.2 million/ml	23.9 million/ml
Motility	23% active 15% sluggish 62% non-motile	55% active 19% sluggish 26% non-motile	63% active 16% sluggish 21% non-motile
Morphology	18% normal	62% normal	66% normal
Vitality	45% live	63% live	69% live

My wife wouldn't respond to my phone calls or letters for a few months, but by June 2006, my results were so amazing, she couldn't ignore me. She moved back home at the end of June, and by September we were delighted to discover she was pregnant.

Thank you so much,

Jim Brown, London UK

Ingredients

Maca

Maca is used by indigenous cultures in South America to enhance fertility, boost the sex drive and increase energy levels.

Scientists at the Universidad Peruana Cayetano Heredia in Peru found that Maca increased semen volume by 31%, sperm count by 34% and increased sperm motility by 108%!

Asian Ginseng

Asian Ginseng boosts sperm concentrations and increases sperm quality and survival rate, increasing the chances of the sperm to reach the egg.

At the University of Rome, medics found that Asian ginseng increased sperm count, improved motility and free testosterone levels. Other studies found that panax ginseng increased semen volume by 23% and increased sperm concentrations in patients with oligospermia.

Asian Ginseng was also reported by the Chungnam National University Medical School to improve erectile function. In Korea, Scientists found that Asian Ginseng increases the survival rate of sperm and improves sperm quality.

Saw Palmetto

Saw Palmetto assists the healthy flow of sperm through the male reproductive system and frees up bound testosterone, has an anti-inflammatory effect on the prostate.

Surgeons at University of Chicago Pritzker School of Medicine found that Saw Palmetto reduced lower urinary tract symptoms in men by as much as 50%

Ginger

Ginger helps to improve sperm motility and increase sperm count. In many cultures, it is used as an aphrodisiac, as it improves circulation to the male genitals.

Researchers at the King Saud University in Saudi Arabia found that Ginger taken with Bok Choy (Chinese Cabbage) and Almonds increased sperm motility and sperm count safely.

Sarsaparilla

Sarsaparilla is used by indigenious people in South America for increasing energy, and sexual impotence. It is rich in plant steroids which can be transformed into testosterone.

Sarsaparilla is also used in Chinese Medicine as a sexual stimulant.

Horny Goat Weed

Horny Goat Weed has been used for hundreds of years by the Chinese to restore testosterone levels, boost the libido in men, and treat premature ejaculation and impotence.

Horny goat weed also improves the circulation, which means an increased circulation of blood, nutrients, oxygen and hormones to the reproductive organs.

Muira Puama

Muira Puama is also known as "Potency Wood", it has been used by Amazonian people to increase sexual arousal in men and it has the effect of reducing body fat percentage and increasing lean muscle mass.

Researchers at the Universidade Federaldo Rio Grande do Sul found that muira puama was effective in treating anxiety, a common cause of low sex drive in men, and erectile dysfunction.

How To Use FertilPlus For Men

Take one capsule, 3 times a day with meals. Because it takes the male reproductive system 90 days to produce new sperm, you will need to take FertilPlus For Men for at least 3 or 4 months before you start seeing results.

To double the effectiveness of FertilPlus for men, combine it with the Body Cleanse Kit. Body cleansing will clear excess toxins and xenoestrogen chemicals which may be responsible for lowering male sex drive, damaging sperm and sperm production.

AlkaGreens Plus can supply you with additional nutrients required to produce strong, healthy sperm.

If you have a sperm morphology or sperm vitality problems, combine FertilPlus For Men with an antioxidant such as AntioxiPlus.

Frequently Asked Questions

Question: Does FertilPlus For Men contain yohimbe?

Answer: No, it does not contain yohimbe.

Question: I'm having problems in maintaining an erection, especially when my partner is ovulating. Any recommendations?

Answer: Stress is a common cause of erectile dysfunction and the stress of trying to conceive has been cited by experts to be as harmful to the body as the stress of bereavement. Stress management or counseling can help you cope with stress, or an excellent alternative is to listen to Quantum Relaxation once a day.

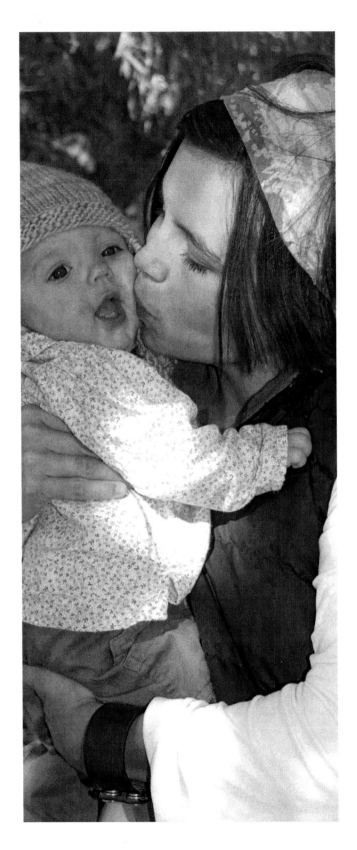

FertilPlus For Women is a herbal blend that balances the hormones, regulates ovulation and menstruation. The ingredients of FertilPlus For Women are also scientifically proven – by doctors, scientists and medical researchers – to increase fertility by up to 330%

FertilPlus For Women

Like all of our remedies, FertilPlus For Women contains only organic and wildcrafted ingredients, and is designed to:

- Balance the hormones and increase ovulation by increasing the release of progesterone, the hormone required for ovulation to take place

- Stimulate the endocrine system which contains all the glands responsible for fertility and hormone balance

- Increase the average number of days in the Luteal Phase with basal temperatures of over 37 degrees by 42%

- Reduce the symptoms of PMS in just after 3 months

- Protect against aging and DNA damage. This is particularly helpful for women who are over 35, or those exposed to toxicity over a long period of time

When Artificial Insemination & IVF Failed
FertilPlus Got Us Pregnant

My name is Liz Arnheim and I live in Pretoria, South Africa. I am 32 years old and had been trying to conceive for 5 years.

We both went through medical tests. My husband's sperm count was said to be excellent. In my case, the first test I took was to check if the fallopian tubes were blocked, and they were not blocked. The second test was the ovulation, and the results were normal. The last diagnosis was that I have fibroids outside the uterus, and that shouldn't be a problem.

We tried artificial insemination 3 times, but that failed, so we started IVF last year. While going through the process, the clinic's staff members were friendly. At the first trial of IVF, the doctors knew that the quality of eggs was poor, and that the zona of the egg was also very hard, thus made it hard to hatch. (Out of ten eggs, only one was better) As a result, implantation did not take place. This was not explained to us during the process.

At the second trial, the eggs were of good quality we were told. (Out of 11 eggs 5 were good, and the best 3 were implanted). None of them hatched.

During the IVF process, I felt stressed, energy drained, tired and I had a deep emotional burden after the negative results. I think this happened because the process sounded too real, especially after the Embryo Transfer.

I also felt that the people at the IVF clinic were trying to avoid my calls after blood test because the results were negative.

I wanted to do the liver, colon and kidney detox after the heavy IVF treatment. I got hold of your product by luck when I was searching for cleansing products on Internet. I read Amina's words on the programme and decided to give it a try. I was sure that it was worth trying while we are waiting for our third IVF treatment in September.

I placed my first order on 02 February 2008. It consisted of FertilPlus and the Body Cleanse Kit. I also placed a second order of Fertil Plus for men on 10 May 2008. My husband agreed to take Fertil plus to maximize our chances of conceiving.

After taking FertilPlus, I had a feeling that there was a hormonal balance taking place because my periods were less painful. Then, after 8 weeks, I missed my period and my breasts became large and sensitive. I suspected I was pregnant but after so many disappointments I didn't want to say anything until I got a positive pregnancy test.

When the test came out positive, we were very happy. The feeling cannot be expressed in words!

I am 7 weeks now. I will be going for my first sonar on Thursday 24th July. I hope all is good. I will try to eat properly, and I'll take AlkaGreens Plus for the nutritional benefits, and rest well and give good energy to the little one in the womb.

So, after 2 failed IVFs, we decided to try fertil plus. We have been taking the capsules for 8 weeks and we just found out that we are 6 weeks pregnant. It's all thanks to you and your good products.

I recommended your products to two friends in Namibia. One received her order already. I will keep on recommending your products to the friends who are dealing with fertility problems because I want them to be happy as I am.

Liz Arnheim, 32, Pretoria, South Africa

FertilPlus is also designed to:

- Assist fetal development and protect the fetus from toxicity

- Provide nutrients required for a healthy pregnancy, including Vitamin B12, folic acid, choline, and iron

- Boost energy levels, and increase the libido in women with a low sex drive

- Support the central nervous system and has antidepressant qualities, helping you prepare mentally and emotionally for conception

- Help the body to deal with both mentally and physically stressful situations

Ingredients

Chaste Tree

Chaste Tree is used to balance the hormones and increase ovulation by increasing the release of progesterone, the hormone required for ovulation to take place. Also known as Chasteberry, Doctors at Stanford University School of Medicine found that it could increase progesterone levels by an average of 56% and increase the average number of days in the Luteal Phase with basal temperatures of over 37 degrees by 42%

Researchers at Basel University, Switzerland found that the herb PMS symptoms by 42.5%

over a period of 3 menstrual cycles, and double-blind placebo-controlled studies have proven that Chaste Tree contains compounds beneficial for regulating menstruation.

93% of women in one study noticed a decrease of PMS symptoms after talking Chaste Tree for just 3 months.

An Australian Researcher at the University of Queensland noted that Chaste Tree is sometimes used by Professional Practitioners to help women avoid miscarriage.

Green Tea

A 2006 double blind, placebo-controlled study carried out by Stanford University of Medicine found that mixing Green Tea extract with Chaste Tree and other vitamins and minerals normalized menstrual cycles in women with both long and short cycles, and resulted in 26% of the women becoming pregnant (compared to just 10% in the placebo group) making it a 260% increase in fertility!

Another 2004 study which contained Green Tea and Chaste Tree extracts resulted in 33% of the women becoming pregnant (and none of the women in the placebo group managed to conceive.)

The Epigallocatechin Gallate in the Green Tea extract was reported in the Food Chemical Toxicology Journal to assist fetal development, as it protected animal fetus from toxicity.

Dong Quai

The Department of Obstetrics and Gynecology, Kwong Wah Hospital, Hong Kong reported use of Dong Quai to help infertile women to conceive.

Dong Quai is used in Chinese Medicine for at least 2000 years to treat female reproductive problems including infertility, frequent miscarriage, ovarian function disorders, uterine cramping, fibroids, endometriosis, ovarian cysts, PMT, painful periods, heavy periods and a lack of periods.

Dong Quai is rich in plant estrogens (phytoestrogens) which help to bring the body back into hormonal balance. It is also a good source of Vitamin B12, folic acid, choline, and iron.

Black Cohosh

Black Cohosh helps to balance estrogen levels and relieve menstrual complaints. A 2002 Biomedical Pharmacotherapy report showed that women talking a mixture of Black Cohosh and Dong Quai reduced menstrual symptoms by 54%.

Unlike many estrogenic substances, Black Cohosh is safe for women with estrogen-related problems such as endometriosis and fibroids, as it does not stimulate endometrial tissue.

Black Cohosh also has anti inflammatory and antioxidant benefits and protects against aging and DNA damage. This is particularly helpful for women who are over 35 or who have been exposed to toxicity.

Muira Puama

Muira Puama has been used by indigenous cultures in South America for aphrodisiac purposes and this has been backed up by the The Institute of Sexology in Paris, which found that 65% of women with a low sex drive who took a blend of Muira Puama reported an increased libido.

In the USA, herbalists use Muira Puama to ease menstrual disorders such as PMS, menstrual crams and to increase fertility. Muira Puama supports the central nervous system and has antidepressant qualities, helping you prepare mentally and emotionally for conception.

Siberian Ginseng

Has been used in Chinese Medicine to help the body to deal with both mentally and physically stressful situations, and to boost energy levels. It stimulates the endocrine system which contains all the glands responsible for fertility and hormone balance.

Siberian Ginseng has anti-aging properties and is particularly useful for older women and it has been widely used as an aphrodisiac and as a general fertility tonic for both men and women. Siberian Ginseng also stimulates the flow of blood to the reproductive organs, and has been used to improve uterine muscles and boost the chances of successful implantation after conception.

How To Take FertilPlus For Women

Take one capsule with meals, 3 times a day. To double the effect of FertilPlus For Women, combine with the Body Cleansing Kit.

Frequently Asked Questions

Question: Since taking FertilPlus For Women, I've been having trouble sleeping. What' should I do?

Answer: This is because it contains Siberian Ginseng, which increases your energy levels. While this is the most gentle of the ginsengs, some women are extra-sensitive, and find they are getting too much of an energy boost in the evening - exactly when they don't need it!

If you're sensitive to Siberian Ginseng, take your last capsule before 3pm, with a mid-afternoon snack, such as a piece of fruit, or AlkaGreens Plus.

Question: I have noticed a change in my cycle since taking FertilPlus For Women. Why is this?

Answer: This is normal, as your hormones are rebalancing themselves, so your next few cycles may be slightly longer, shorter, heavier or lighter than usual.

Question: I am very sensitive to herbs and I am worries about side effects. Can I still take FertilPlus?

Answer: Yes - the suggested doses are average doses and are safe to take. However, if you are particularly sensitive, here's an alternative way to take your herbal remedy.

Take one capsule a day (with breakfast) for one week, and see how you feel. If are not feeling sensitive to the herbs, increase your dosage to 2 capsules a day (one with breakfast and one with lunch). Continue taking 2 capsules for another week.

For some women - particularly those who are very petite, or have little body fat, this may be enough to help you conceive.

However, if you wish to increase to the recommended amount, wait another week until your body has become accustomed to the herbs and increase your intake 3 capsules a day (one with breakfast, one with lunch and one with your mid-afternoon snack, before 3pm.)

Please note: If you are used to taking herbal remedies, or are not sensitive to herbs, start taking FertiPlus 3 times a day.

Question: I have had several rounds of IVF, which have not worked out, and I am ready to try natural remedies. Do I need to do a cleanse first?

Answer: If you have been exposed to any kind of drug that affects your reproductive system (directly or indirectly), we recommend you do a cleanse to get rid of the drug residues in your body.

This also applies if you have taken contraceptives, fertility drugs, or medication for condition such as endometriosis, fibroids, or PCOS.

Question: Can I take FertilPlus For Women with fertility drugs?

Answer: We don't recommend you mix herbal remedies with drugs, without the express permission of the medical professional who prescribed the drugs.

Question: Can I mix FertilPlus For Women With Acupuncture?

Answer: Acupuncture is excellent for increasing your chances of conceiving, and we have found many scientific studies that prove its effectiveness. It is safe to mix FertilPlus For Women with acupuncture.

Note: If you would like to get the benefits of acupuncture, but you are terrified of needles, use the acupressure techniques in the Chinese Fertility DVD.

Question: I have blocked fallopian tubes - can FertilPlus for women help?

Answer: Blocked fallopian tubes are a condition that results in sperm not being able to reach the egg - or a partially blocked tube that will not let a fertilized egg reach the uterus.

FertilPlus for women cannot unblock fallopian tubes. Instead we recommend you use the blocked fallopian tube kit.

Question: Do you have any recommendations for mature mothers?

Yes, we have prepared a Mature Mothers Kit, which includes a Body Cleansing, FertilPlus For Women, AlkaGreens Plus and AntioxiPlus.

Question: I have taken FertilPlus For Women and I'm now pregnant. Should I continue taking it?

Answer: Congratulations! FertilPlus For Women has now done its job, and you no longer need to take it.

We recommend you switch to AlkaGreens Plus to provide you and your growing baby with the nutrients required for a healthy pregnancy.

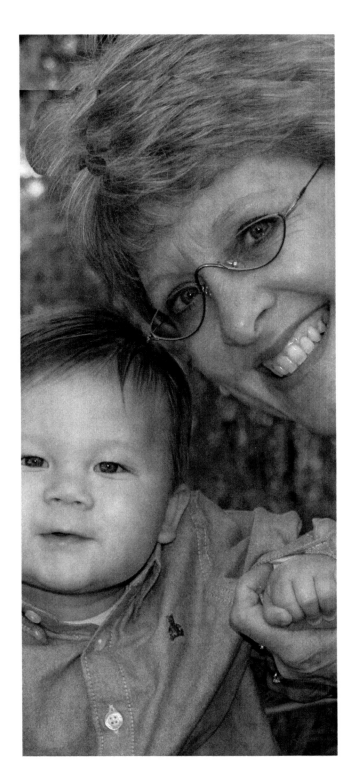

IIf you are aged 40 or over and you want to get pregnant fast, try the Mature Mother's Kit, our organic and wildcrafted solution for improving egg quality, regulating menstruation, ovulation and increasing your fertility by 660%

Mature Mother's Kit

We have put together what we have found works best for mature women who are trying to conceive:

1. Body cleanse for fertility, consisting of:

   - Colon Cleansing Kit

   - Liver Cleansing Kit

   - Kidney Cleansing Kit

   - Toxin Cleansing Kit

2. 4 month supply of FertilPlus For Women

3. 4 month supply of FertilPlus For Men (optional)

4. 4 month supply of AlkaGreens Plus

5. 4 month supply of AntioxiPlus

6. Quantum Relaxation CD

Blocked Fallopian Tubes

Having blocked fallopian tubes does not mean you need surgery to conceive.

Blocked Fallopian Tubes

7 Steps to Unblocking Your Fallopian Tubes
By Shola Oslo

Have you been diagnosed with blocked fallopian tubes, and are you looking for a natural alternative that will help you get pregnant fast? If so, please keep reading.

I'm a kinesiologist who has developed a 7-step process for unblocking blocked fallopian tubes, and helping women to get pregnant in the shortest time possible. I've had great success with my own private clients, and I'd like to share with you how I helped these women to get pregnant, and how you can overcome tubal infertility without surgery.

Step 1: Herbal Tampons & Herbal Douches - The key step in the process involves using herbal tampons to introduce a powerful herbal decoction to the reproductive organs and the fallopian tubes. The herbs in the tampons are designed to kill any infections left in the fallopian tubes, break up adhesions and scar tissues, and soothe swollen tissues.

The herbal tampons are used every night after menstruation and before ovulation, and the douche is used in the morning to cleanse the reproductive organs of any debris loosened up by the herbal tampons.

Step 2: Herbal Capsules For Blocked Fallopian Tubes - Step 2 involves taking a blend of herbs that strengthen the actions of the herbal tampons. This herbal blend is 100% organic, and is designed to help the immune system fight off infections that can block the tubes, as well as increase the fertility and boost the sex drive.

All of my clients who want to get pregnant with blocked fallopian tubes take herbal capsules 3 times a day, in addition to the herbal tampons.

Step 3: Chinese Fertility Massage - The fertility massage helps to open up the reproductive organs, as it can break up adhesions, soften scar tissue and improve the health of the fallopian tubes and uterus.

For best results, I ask my clients to perform this massage while wearing the herbal tampon.

Step 4: Fertility Yoga - The fertility yoga positions my clients practice help to overcome tubal fertility as they stretch the organs, and indirectly soften scar tissue. Some of the yoga positions are designed to increase the flow of blood, oxygen and nutrients to the pituitary gland (which governs the reproductive hormones), while other positions help the reproductive organs.

To increase the effectiveness of the herbal tampons, my clients perform the yoga every morning, before taking the tampon out.

Step 5: Total Body Cleansing For Fertility - The body cleansing for fertility program helps the body to get rid of toxins that damage the fertility, or cause the reproductive organs to become inflamed or infected. It includes a colon cleanse, liver cleanse, kidney cleanse, heavy metal cleanse, and a parasite cleanse. All of these cleanses support the liver in recycling old hormones and maintaining the balance of hormones, and they can prevent conditions such as fibroids, endometriosis, PCOS, and PID, which can affect the fertility.

Another benefit of the body cleanse is that it can double the effectiveness of any herbal remedy you take. This means you will shorten the time it takes you to get pregnant by approximately 50% - if you decide to carry out this important step.

Step 6: Stress Management & Relaxation - It's important to manage your stress levels while trying to conceive, as stress can prevent you from getting pregnant. This is because when you're stressed, you release a hormone called cortisol, which can affect the balance of other hormones in the body (such as estrogen and progesterone).

When you're stressed, you're more likely to experience spasms in the fallopian tubes, or any other part of the reproductive organs, which can prevent sperm from reaching the egg, or it can prevent successful implantation.

The fastest way to manage stress is by listening to an audio CD, which puts your brain into a relaxation state. Once the brain waves have slowed down, the body will relax and be more conducive to conception.

Step 7: Nutritional Optimization - One of the fastest ways to boost the fertility is by changing the diet. I find that my clients get the best results by increasing their intake of raw fruits and vegetables to 9 portions a day. Eating fruits and vegetables in their raw form helps you to access the nutrients in the foods, increases your intake of antioxidants and alkalizes the body.

Antioxidants can help reverse the effects of free radicals and make the reproductive organs younger and healthier. They have also been proven to improve egg quality. To get the maximum amount of antioxidants in your daily intake, I recommend mixing an antioxidant into your juice every morning.

Alkalizing foods help to neutralize excessively acidic cervical mucus, which can be very hostile to sperm, and prevent conception. These foods also support your detoxification, as they create an internal environment in which bacteria and viruses cannot survive. The best way to eat a large quantity of nutrient dense foods is with an alkaline mix, which an contain a number of superfood fruits and vegetables, and can be available in a form that can be added to juice, water or smoothies.

Do the 7 steps for unblocking fallopian tubes work? The answer is yes - in the past 12 months, I have had success rates of 73%, and practitioners of Traditional Chinese Medicine at Shenzhen Municipal Hospital of Traditional Chinese Medicine in Guangdong, China, where doctors were achieving 82.22% success rates using a similar process.

Case Studies:

Jenny Conceived In 5 Months With Blocked Tubes And A History of Chlamydia & PID

Jenny was 38 years old when she first visited, and had a history of Chlamydia infections and pelvic inflammatory disease. She'd been trying to conceive for 4 years and had had an HSG, which confirmed that both of her fallopian tubes were blocked. Her husband's sperm count and motility was normal, so we focussed on her.

She was lucky to have a very supportive partner who learned the massage techniques and acupressure points, and performed the yoga with her every morning. It only took her 5 months to conceive.

Lola Finally Became Pregnant... At Age 46 (With Methods After $160,000 of IVF Failed)

Lola was 46 and had spent over $160,000 on IVF treatments over the past 3 years. She was extremely stressed and toxic when she came to my clinic and I managed to convince her to spend 4 weeks on a body cleansing, healthy eating, relaxation and exercise program before attempting to unblock her tubes. She lost weight in the first 4 weeks and doubled her energy levels.

When she started to use the herbal tampons, massage and yoga, it only took her 2 months

Sarah Became Pregnant In 4 Months
With One Fallopian Tube

Sarah was 29 and had an ectopic pregnancy, which resulted in a salpingectomy – this is the surgical removal of a fallopian tube. Her remaining fallopian tube was also blocked, and she didn't want to risk surgery on the tube, as she was worried about scarring and future ectopic pregnancies.

Sarah followed the 7 steps and became pregnant after 4 months.

Caryn Got Pregnant In 3 Months...
With Salpingitis & Frequent Yeast Infections

Caryn's was 37 and had salpingitis, which is the inflammation of the fallopian tubes. She had also had frequent yeast infections, which she had passed on to her partner and he'd pass on to her. I gave both of them DidaClear, which is a herbal remedy for yeast infections, and they both did the cleansing program.

Caryn also followed the rest of the 7 steps, and reported feeling better in just 5 weeks. In total, it took her 3 months to conceive.

Lynne Took 4 Months To Conceive
(And Her Husband Had A Low Sperm Count Too)

Lynne was 40 and was a smoker who had also had scar tissue on her fallopian tubes from a previous surgery to open them up. The first thing we worked on was to stop smoking, and increase her intake of nutrients, then we started the 7 steps.

Her husband also took FertilPlus for Men, as his sperm count was lower than average. It took Lynne just 4 months to conceive, and I'm pleased to say she no longer smokes.

Miriam Took Only 6 Weeks To Get Pregnant

Miriam was 35 and diagnosed with blocked fallopian tubes, and had been trying to conceive for the past 3 years. She was very committed to following the 7-step program, and it only took her 6 weeks to unblock her fallopian tubes and conceive.

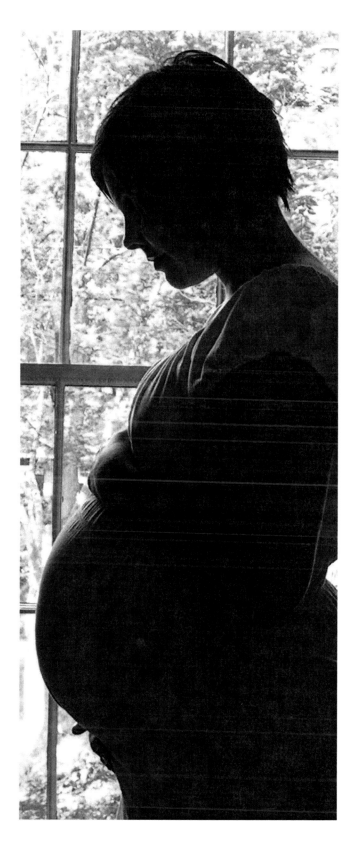

To assist you in unblocking your fallopian tubes naturally, we have put together a Blocked Fallopian Tube Kit, which consists of all the products recommended for unblocking your tubes, as well as additional recommendations for increasing your chances of conceiving in the next 6 months.

Blocked Fallopian Tube Kit

The Blocked Fallopian Tubes Kit consists of:

Fallopen Herbal Tampon Mix - a blend of herbs that kill infections, reduce inflammation in the fallopian tubes, reduce scarring, increase the circulation of blood, nutrients and oxygen to the fallopian tubes, and help to loosen up adhesions and scar tissue.

Chamomile Cleanse Herbal Douche Mix - a blend of herbs that wash the vagina and pelvic organs of debris loosed up by the herbal tampons, and kill any remaining infections, while helping to restore the vagina's natural flora

FalloClear Herbal Capsules - a herbal blend of capsules that support the action of the herbal tampons by stimulating the circulation to the pelvic organs and fallopian tubes, and contains enzymes that break up adhesions and scar tissue.

Fertility Massage DVD - contains the fallopian tube massage for breaking up scar tissue and opening the fallopian tubes, and a regular fertility massage you can practice any time of the month, for relaxing and stimulating the uterus, fallopian tubes and ovaries.

Fertility Yoga DVD - contains a full fertility yoga routine for balancing the hormones, stretching, toning and opening up the pelvic organs, relaxing the mind, body and spirit and an exercise you and your partner can do together to harmonize your energies, making conception easier.

Quantum Relaxation CD - the exact CD I give to my clients to stimulate a deep level of relaxation. It works using sounds that stimulate the brain waves, and gently alter the frequencies of your brain waves to match that of relaxation and regeneration.

Blocked Fallopian Tubes Book - a full explanation of everything you need to do to unblock your fallopian tubes and become pregnant. It also contains advice on herbal remedies for male and female fertility, diet and nutrition advice for men and women, how to time sex for conception and sexual positions and sex tips for conception.

Fast Start CD - I talk you through everything you need to do to get started, and provide you with a handy summary card for easy reference.

If you would like to increase your chances of conceiving and follow the exact 7-step procedure Shola Oslo recommends, you will need to add:

• Body Cleanse Kit

• Ultra Nutrition Plus Kit

to your order.

For more information on how to use the items in the Blocked Fallopian Tube Kit, please refer to the book that came with your kit.

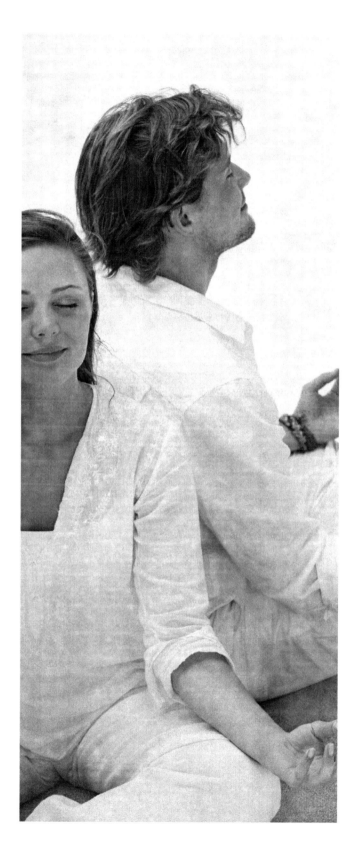

Fertility yoga consists of the asanas (or positions) that nourish the reproductive organs, endocrine system and brain, while opening up the pelvic organs and gently exercising the uterus, ovaries and fallopian tubes.

Fertility Yoga

Fertility yoga can stretch the internal organs and accelerate the process of breaking up adhesions and scar tissue, while opening up the reproductive organs and preparing the body mentally, physically and emotionally for conception and pregnancy.

- Increases the energy levels, by releasing pent up energy levels for positive uses, such as starting new life

- Relieves stress, calms the mind of anxiety and promotes relaxation

- Increases the flow of blood, lymph (and therefore oxygen and nutrients) to the brain, organs and endocrine system.

- Relaxes the muscles — both internal and external,

- Calms the sympathetic nervous system, allowing the reproductive organs to be relaxed, supple and well-nourished for conception.

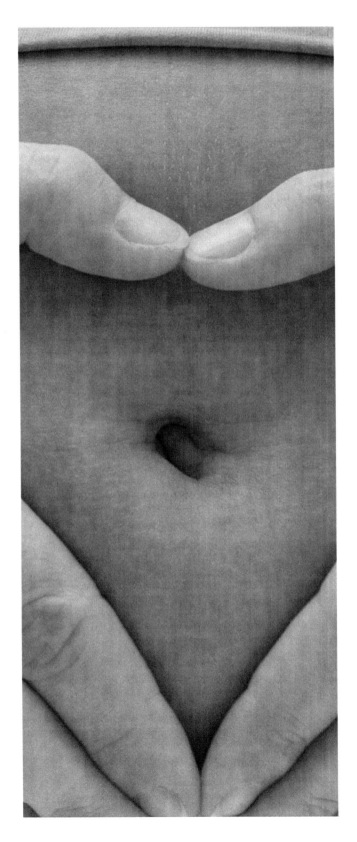

This fertility massage uses techniques from Traditional Chinese Medicine and was developed to improve the health of the reproductive organs, break up adhesions and unblock fallopian tubes, and combines deep tissue massage, with acupressure.

Fertility Massage

This fertility massage also:

- Loosens up congestion, energy and physical blockages in the reproductive system

- Stimulates and strengthens the internal organs,

- Improves circulation of blood, oxygen and lymph to the reproductive organs,

- Stimulates the digestion, and removal of toxins from the body

- Repositions a displaced uterus into its correct position in the body and stimulates the muscles that support the pelvis and reproductive organs

- Balances the hormones, regulating the menstrual cycle, and can relieve symptoms of hormone-aggravated conditions such as PCOS, endometriosis, fibroids, and PreMenstrual Tension

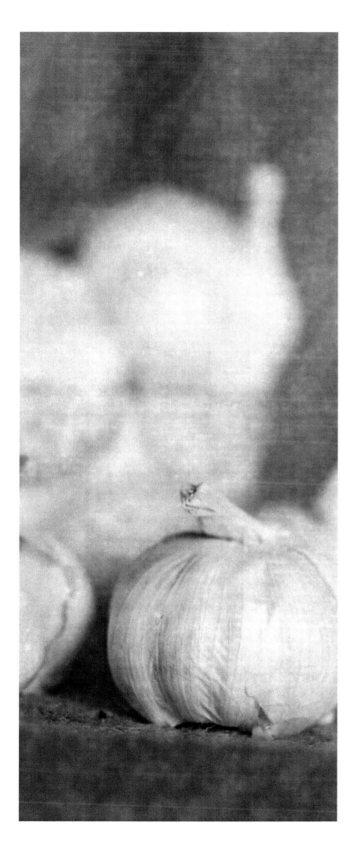

Herbal tampons are a safe way to introduce medicinal herbs directly into the fallopian tubes to kill infections, reduce inflammation and loosen up scar tissue and adhesions.

Fallopen Herbal Tampon Mix

The active ingredients of the herbs work directly on the tissues of the pelvic organs, and have the following effects:

- Reducing inflammation in the fallopian tubes

- Killing infections, bacteria, viruses yeast and fungus

- Strenghening the immune system, to enable the body to fight conditions such as Pelvic Inflammatory Disease

- Speeding up healing of damaged fallopian tubes

- Softening and breaking up adhesions and scar tissue

- Keeping the delicate tissues of the reproductive tract healthy and moist.

The herbs in Fallopen have been finely ground, to enable the active ingredients to be easily released upon contact with hot water.   Fallopen Herbal Tampon Mix needs to be combined with the other 7 steps for best results.

Ingredients

Calendula

Calendula flowers have been used in European medicine for nearly a thousand of years to reduce inflammation, heal broken skin and relieve menstrual cramps and spasms.

Calendula was found by a Dermatovenereological Clinic to speed up the healing of skin wounds, as it stimulates the flow of blood to the organs, and biologists at the American University of Beirut confirmed that the herb reduces inflammation and swelling.

It is rich in flavioids, which protect the cells from free radicals, unstable molecules which that accelerate the agining of tissues. Researchers at Nihon University found four compounds in calendula that protect against inflammation and cancer. Calendula also kills fungus, bacteria and viruses, protecting your organs from the infections that cause Pelvic Inflammatory Disease and damage fallopian tubes.

Goldenseal

Goldenseal has been traditionally used in Native American medicine to heal skin problems, and was adopted by Americans in the early 20th century to treat menstrual problems in women. it is a powerful natural disinfectant, and is used by herbalists to disinfect cuts and skin wounds.

Goldenseal is rich in berberine, which helps to fight infection, and was confirmed by Pharmacists at the University of Illinois at Chicago to kill bacteria, candida, viruses and parasites. Berberine has also been scientifically proven to increase the flow of blood to the tiny blood vessels, which increases the supply of nutrients and oxygens to the delicate fallopian tubes. It's has been used successfully in TCM to stimulate the flow of blood to the pelvic area and uterus.

Goldenseal has been scientifically proven to strengthen the immune system, and is a common herb used for reducing inflammation caused by infections, and disinfecting cuts and broken skin.

It reduces inflammation in the mucus membranes - these are the tissues that line the genitals, reproductive tract and fallopian tubes. Studies have confirmed that goldenseal increases the flow of mucus in the mucous membranes, which is excellent for maintaining the health and flexibiity of the fallopian tubes. It is a common ingredient in natural treatments for vulvovaginitis, and similar conditions relating to the female reproductive system.

Animal studies at the University of Rome La Sapienza, Pharmacologists found that goldenseal contained active components that acted as a relaxant, which can be useful in women who suffer cramps and spasms.

Garlic

Garlic has been used for thousands of years as a food and medicine all over the world, and is a common ingredient in herbal douches for getting rid of infections in the vagina, uterus and fallopian tubes.

Garlic is a powerful antioxidant that destroys free radicals, and protect the cells from damage and genetic mutation. It can strengthen the immune system, and help the body to fight infection, as it is rich in allicin, a compound that kills viruses, fungus and bacteria. In fact, researchers at Sejong University reported that allicin killed both yeasts and fungus, and mentioned candida as one of the microbes it was effective against. It's antibiotic effects are so powerful that the Shiraz University of Medical Sciences recognized that garlic extract could kill infections resistant to multiple drugs.

Garlic has very powerful antimicrobial and antibiotic effects, due to its high sulphur content, and was recognized by the American University to help the body get rid of harmful foreign substances, such as heavy metals. (The Institute of Chemical Biology, Kolkata found that garlic was even effective against of arsenic toxicity!)

Scientists at the Liverpool John Moores University found that garlic prevents platelets from aggregating, which has the effect of reducing blood clots and the formation of scabs and scar tissue. Biologists at the

Universidad Nacional de Luján found that garlic prevented red blood cells from clumping together abnormally in the presence of bacteria, an antibody or an allergen.

Red Clover

Red Clover has been traditionally used to reduce inflammation, purify the blood, improve the circulation and help the body to expel excess fluid.

Herbalists have used red clover to break up scar tissue, and it is a common ingredient in herbal treatments for scars and inflammation as it contains compounds that can break down the proteins that form scar tissues. Researchers from the Biotechnology and Biological Sciences Research Council reported that red clover contained enzymes that had a mild effect of breaking down proteins.

The Georg-August-University found an isoflavone genistein (plant estrogen) in red clover, which also had antioxidant activities. It was also identified by the University of Illinois College of Pharmacy to contain plant estrogens that were recognized by estrogen receptors, making this herb an excellent for its use in helping the uterus build a healthy lining.   Plant estrogens are weak estrogens that attach to estrogen receptors and block the cells from using stronger, more harmful forms of estrogens such as xenoestrogens.

Corydalis Root

Corydalis root is used in Traditional Chinese Medicine to relieve pain, treat menstrual disorders, and stimulate the flow of blood to the uterus and fallopian tubes.

Traditional Chinese Medicine views blocked fallopian tubes as a problem mostly related to stagnant blood energies, and treats this condition with herbs that invigorate the blood, such as corydalis root. This is because corydalis root is also used as a cleanser, and researchers at Gazi University, identified 33 compounds in corydalis that killed fungus and viruses.

Corydalis root has also been used in Chinese Medicine to calm the nervous system and relieve pain related to menstruation and uterine spasms. Pharmacists at the Second Military Medical University identified ten separate alkaloids in corydalis. Alkaloids are natural compounds that can be used for a numer of phamacological effects, for example, pain relief and anaesthesia.

Astralgus Root

Astralgus root has been used in Traditional Chinese medicine to protect the body from disease, improve circulation and boost the immune system. It is also used to treat wounds, making it ideal for topical treatment of damaged tissues in the female reproductive tract. Astralgus kills bacteria and viruses, and is a common ingredient in Chinese medicine decoctions for treating female reproductive disorders.

Researchers at Seoul National University identified two new saponins in astralgus. Saponins are antioxidants that stimulate the immune system, and protect against microbes, fungus, protozoa, and viruses. Doctors at the Queen Elizabeth Hospital, Hong Kong found that astralgus restored the immune system, which is particularly helpful if you have had a history of infections or endometriosis. It was also listed by Biochemists at Xinzhou Teachers University as an important herb for protecting the DNA. In addition to this, the polysaccharides in astralgus were found by Lanzhou University to promote the activity of macrophages - immune cells that remove debris and waste material from the body.

Sapoinins also have anti inflammatory effects, and the anti-inflammatory effects of astralgus were confirmed by biologists at Ajou University in January 2008. This is particularly beneficial for women whose tubes are blocked due to Pelvic Inflammatory Disease or infections. Because astralgus also helps to remove excess fluids from the body, it can be helpful in removing hydrosalpinges as well as inflammation of the uterus and fallopian tubes.

Ligusticum

Ligusticum is a medicinal herb used in Traditional Chinese Medicine to improve the circulation of blood and remove stagnant energy, which the Chinese believe to be the cause of blocked fallopian tubes.

According to Traditional Chinese Medicine, the herb warms the uterus by improving the supply of blood to the pelvic organs (including the fallopian tubes) and reduces swelling in the area.

Chemists at Yunnan University found that it contains ferulic acid, an antioxidant that can protect against DNA damage and cell aging, and chlorogenic acid, which kills bacteria, viruses and fungus, and can protect against tumors. Researchers at Tsinghua University, Beijing found that ligusticum contained caffeic acid - an antioxidant that kills fungus, reduces inflammation and protects the skin and mucus membranes from disease. The Macao Polytechnic Institute specifically identified ligusticum as one of the herbs that demonstrated greatest DNA protective effect.

In animal studies, ligusticum was idenfified by the Yong Loo Lin School of Medicine to have a slight progestogen effect, which balances out the estrogenic effect of the red clover.

Dong Quai

Dong Quai has been used for thousands of years in Traditional Chinese Medicine to treat menstrual disorders such as premenstrual syndrome, uterine cramps, irregular menstrual cycles and infertility in women. It is also used for the treatment of fallopian tube obstructions by the Shenzhen Municipal Hospital In Guangdong, China.

It contains antispasmodic properties to prevent spasms and cramps in the uterus, allowing the uterine muscles to relax, and enable the flow of blood, nutrients and lymphatic tissues to nourish the reproductive tract. This is particularly helpful for women whose tubes are closed due to muscle spasms.

A 2007 study carried out at the Shaanxi Normal University found that Dong Quai was rich in antioxidants (antioxidants prevent tissue damage and can slow down aging), and the polysaccharides in Dong Quai stimulated the immune system, and helped the immune cells to remove dead cell material and waste products, and break down over 100 different types of bacteria.

Dong quai has also been used to prevent clots from forming, and when used on the skin, can stop scabbing and scarring from taking place. This benefit can also apply to the mucus membranes of the fallopian tubes.

How To Use Fallopen

Herbal tampons should not be used during menstruation, but between menstruation and ovulation, and should not be used after ovulation.   Here are the steps involved:

1. Put a teaspoon of the herbal tampon mix into a clean cup or small container, then add a quarter of a cup of boiling water to the herbs and leave to steep for 5 minutes.

1. When the water has cooled, pour the mixture into another cup or container, using a filter or strainer. It is important to use a fine filter, such as a coffee filter, in order to keep the liquid as "clear" as possible.

2. Place a tampon into the strained herbal mixture for about 30 seconds, or until the tampon is completely soaked.

3. Insert the soaked tampon into your vagina. This may be a little more tricky than normal, since the tampon will be wet. (You may wish to practice inserting wet tampons until you're ready to use the herbal tampons.)

You will need to use a light sanitary towel or panty liner with the herbal tampon, as some of the liquid will leak out, especially if you are very active.

It is recommended to use the tampon just before you go to sleep, as lying down will help the herbal tampon mixture to move into the uterus and fallopian tubes.

Practice the Chinese Fertility Massage techniques while wearing the herbal tampon, as this will loosen up adhesions and break up scar tissues. (You can follow along with the fallopian tube massage section of the Chinese Fertility Massage DVD for best results).

You can sleep with the herbal tampon inside you, as the herbs will work more effectively

overnight while you are in your relaxed state. In the morning, simply remove your tampon and douche with Chamomile Cleanse.

Important note:

It's important to observe strict hygiene when preparing, inserting and taking out the tampons, to avoid introducing bacteria from your hands, instruments or surroundings into your pelvic organs. You should wash your hands thoroughly before preparing the tampon and keep the cups or containers sterile, washing them with a good detergent, then giving them a final rinse with boiling water.

Frequently Asked Questions
Question: Should I still try to get pregnant while using the tampon?

Answer: The herbal tampon should be used after menstruation but before ovulation. You do not use the tampons while you are ovulating, so you can still try to get pregnant.

Question: Do I need to use the massage, yoga, and other techniques for the tampons to work?

Answer: All of the women who have conceived using our Blocked Fallopian Tubes kit has followed all 7-steps. We do not recommend you skip any of the 7 steps.

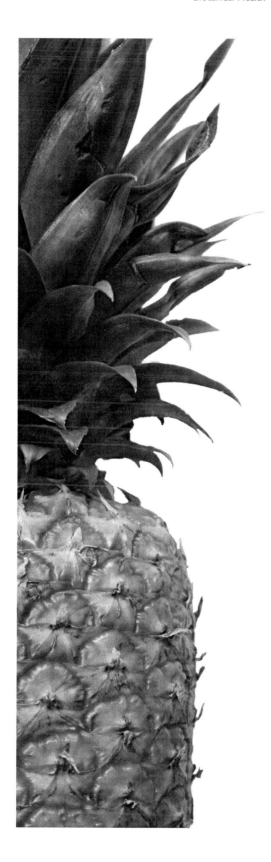

FalloClear allows herbs to reach the fallopian tubes indirectly, via the digestive system, and increase the effectiveness of the herbal tampons, while protecting the body from infections that cause fallopian tubes to become blocked.

FalloClear

FalloClear helps women in opening up their fallopian tubes, increasing the fertility, boosting the immune system, and preparing the female body for conception. It helps to improve fertility by:

- Boosting the immune system and protecting against Pelvic Inflammatory Disease

- Balancing progesterone, LH, FSH and estrogen

- Improving fertility, regulating menstruation and ovulation

- Increasing the sex drive

The capsules are taken every day with meals for at least a month. If you have had a history of recurrent pelvic inflammatory disease, or have had extensive scarring from previous surgeries take FalloClear capsules until you get pregnant.

Ingredients

Tribulus Terrestris

Tribulus terrestris is commonly used in Ayurvedic medicine (a system of Indian medicine used for thousands of years) to improve fertility. It is rich in steroidal saponins, which naturally decrease inflammation, decrease clotting , reduce scar tissues, and repair the skin and mucus membranes. It is also a natural painkiller, which is helpful for women experiencing pain due to blockages or inflammation of the fallopian tubes.

In Chinese Medicine Tribulus terrestris is used for its anti-fungal and antibacterial properties to treat vaginal infections, and infections of the female reproductive organs. A scientific study from the University of Mosul found that the herb killed 11 species of microorganisms, including candida albicans.

Studies have shown that the herbs can stimulate the production of LH and FSH to increase fertility and libido, and a recent study carried out in Valparaiso University confirmed its use for treating sexual dysfunction.

Pineapple Extract

Pineapples have been used for hundreds of years in Asia and South America as a herbal medicine, and is one of the most commonly used herbal medicines in Germany.

Although pineapples are a fruit, they contain a enzyme called bromelain, which breaks up proteins. This natural enzyme can break down abnormal tissues, such as the adhesions that cause fallopian tubes to become blocked.

Bromelain is used in modern medicine to reduce inflammation, and assist the healing of broken tissues following injury or surgery. The Friedrich-Schiller-University found it could be effectively used to stop platelets from aggregating, preventing the formation of clots, which can block fallopian tubes, and it can help to treat painful menstruation.

Studies carried out at a medical facility in Cuba revealed that bromelain prevented tumors from forming, which is good news for women whose tubes are blocked because of endometrial growths.

Chaste Tree

Chaste Tree is mostly used in Chinese Medicine to treat disorders relating to the female reproductive system. It has been used in Western herbal medicine as far back as the 4th Century BC by Hippocrates as an ingredient in a sitz bath to treat diseases of the uterus, and was used in Europe during the Middle Ages for reducing the inflammation of the female reproductive organs.

Chaste Tree balances the female hormones, and is known to lower prolactin levels.

Prolactin is the hormone that stimulates lactation, and prevents conception in women with high prolactin levels.

Pharmacologists at Ege University found that chaste tree had a good level of antioxidant activity, and researchers at the Tokyo University of Pharmacy & Life Science found that chaste tree was rich in flavinoids. Flavoinoids help the body to cope with viruses, and irritants. They also control any allergic reactions, and reduce inflammation, and have been noted to protect the cells from carcinogens and genetic damage.

Chaste Tree can ease pelvic discomfort caused by inflammation or complications due to blocked fallopian tubes, while helping the body to balance its hormone levels naturally.

Green Tea

Green tea has a high concentration of antioxidants called polyphenols, which prevent the cells from damage and mutation. It also helps to stop excess bleeding (of wounds) and promote healing to damaged tissues.

Many studies, including a 2008 study published in the British Journal of Dermatology have indicated that when applied to the skin, the polyphenols in green tea is effective in preventing cell mutation and the formation of growths and tumors, so it is an ideal addition to any formula for relieving blocked fallopian tubes.

FalloClear also contains the following ingredients, which are also present in the Fallopen Herbal Tampon Mix:

- Astragalus Root

- Chaste Tree

- Dong Quai

- Garlic

- Goldenseal

How To Take FalloClear

Taking FalloClear 3 times a day with meals while you're working on unblocking your fallopian tubes can help to accelerate the work of the herbal tampons, especially when combined with massage.

Frequently Asked Questions

Question: Why are some of the ingredients the same as the Fallopen Herbal Tampon Mix?

Answer: We have found that some herbs are so powerful for women with blocked fallopian tubes, that they should be both taken orally and topically (on the skin).

Question: Should I take FalloClear for longer than 30 days?

Answer: If you have had a history of PID or chlamydia, we recommend you take FalloClear every day until you conceive.,

The Chamomile Herbal Cleanse is a douche used to cleanse the pelvic organs of any debris left from the herbal tampons, massage and yoga. It is also designed to kill any remaining infections, while helping to restore the vagina's natural flora

Chamomile Cleanse

The Chamomile cleanse is an important part of the 7-step process for unblocking fallopian tubes, and contains the following cleansing and healing herbs:

Chamomile

Chamomile is an excellent herb to use in a douche, as it been used for thousands of years to treat a number of different conditions, including inflammation, infections, wounds and skin complaints. It is antibacterial, anti-fungal and antiseptic.

Pau D'Arco

Pau d'arco is a less common herb used in douching, but is a common ingredient in herbal remedies for bacterial infections, candida, inflammation, and viral infections. Its addition to a douche means you can e sure of killing any infections that cause Pelvic Inflammatory Disease.

How To Use The Chamomile Cleanse

The instructions for using Chamomile Cleanse are below:

Put 4 teaspoons into a large container (such as a teapot or mixing bowl) and add a liter (about 2 pints) of hot water to the herbs. Leave the mixture to steep for 5 minutes, or until the mixture has cooled.

When the water has cooled, pour the mixture into another cup or container, using a filter or strainer. It is important to use a fine filter, such as a coffee filter, in order to keep the liquid as "clear" as possible.

Put the mixture into a douche bottle or bag.

Stand in the bathtub or shower, and introduce the nozzle of the douche into the vagina, then squeeze the bottle slowly to allow the liquid to flow into the vagina.

If you have a vaginal yeast infection, you may wish to allow the liquids to stay in the vagina for longer, so the herbs can work on killing the infection. If this is the case, you should lie in the bathtub with your hips raised for a few minutes, so the liquid does not spill out.

For optimal hygiene, keep your douche bottle sterile with a good cleaning solution and lots of boiled water.

Frequently Asked Questions

Question: Should I be able to see the scar tissue coming out in the douche?

Answer: The fallopian tubes are about 4 to 5 inches long, but only 0.2 to 0.5 inches in diameter, and any scar tissue will be relatively small, compared to the fallopian tube size.

The 7-step process is designed to stretch, loosen and break up scar tissue over a period of several days, so we do not expect you to find any visible pieces of scar tissue in your douche.

Question: How long should the herbal tampons and douche last?

Answer: They should each last approximately 3 menstrual cycles, if used after menstruation and before ovulation.

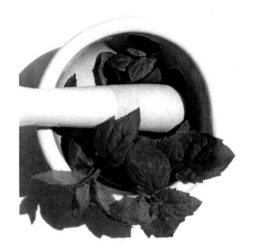

Herbal Remedies

In the past 50 years we have seen a rise in hormone-related health problems, such as fibroids, endometriosis, ovarian cysts, poly cystic breasts, infertility and even some types of breast, ovarian and cervical cancers.

Young girls are experiencing puberty at alarmingly young ages, and women are being diagnosed with these reproductive diseases at a much earlier ages than ever before.

Herbal Remedies For Women

Conditions such as Premenstrual Syndrome, characterized by weight gain, bloating, fatigue, depression, mood swings and tender breasts, are being experienced by increasing amount of women every month - yet is it still not taken seriously as a medical condition.

Why is that? The answer is a lack of hormone balance - in particular, high levels of estrogen, and low levels of progesterone.

Many women have been exposed to synthetic hormones in the form of the contraceptive pill, fertility medications, drugs prescribed for the treatment of fibroids, endometriosis, and PCOS, and in Hormone Replacement Therapy.

Another source of synthetic hormones are xenoestrogens - byproducts of the chemical industry which mimic our natural estrogen, and cause a range of reproductive complaints. Xenoestrogens can be found in exhaust fumes, contaminated water, pesticides sprayed on fruits and vegetables, and in plastics used to store food and water.

Non-commercial sources of meat and dairy products are also affected by these synthetic hormones, as animals are routinely given hormones, antibiotics, drugs and other substances in order to make them grow larger, produce more milk and reach a good selling price.

These chemicals are even in our cleaning products, cosmetics and gardening supplies, along with other harmful chemicals that make reproductive conditions worse, such as dioxins and parabens.

Unfortunately, the human body is ill-equipped to detoxify these chemicals, so they can remain in the human body for years, making conditions such as fibroids and endometriosis worse, and being passed on to future generations through the placenta and via breast milk.

In order to bring conditions such as fibroids and endometriosis under control, it is important to eliminate these sources of synthetic hormones wherever possible.

This means switching from commercial produce and processed foods to fresh organic foods, using natural cleaning products and cosmetics, and avoiding the use of plastics in storing food and water.

 The next step is to detoxify the build up of these chemicals from your tissues, and to strengthen the organs of elimination. This can be done with a total body cleanse, such as the Body Cleanse Kit.

Balancing hormones naturally is of vital importance and herbal remedies designed to raise the progesterone levels naturally should be added to any natural health program for women.

It is also vital to introduce weaker phytoestrogens - plant-based estrogen, that block the synthetic estrogens from causing further damage to your body. Both FibroidClear and EndoClear supply the body with plant-based hormones, and can be taken while doing the body cleanse.

Finally, supporting your natural healing program with a food-based nutrient supplement such as AlkaGreens Plus will give you the vitamins, minerals, phytonutrients, enzymes and amino acids required to heal damaged tissues, reduce inflammation and give you the energy needed to lead a normal, fulfilling life, without adding many calories.

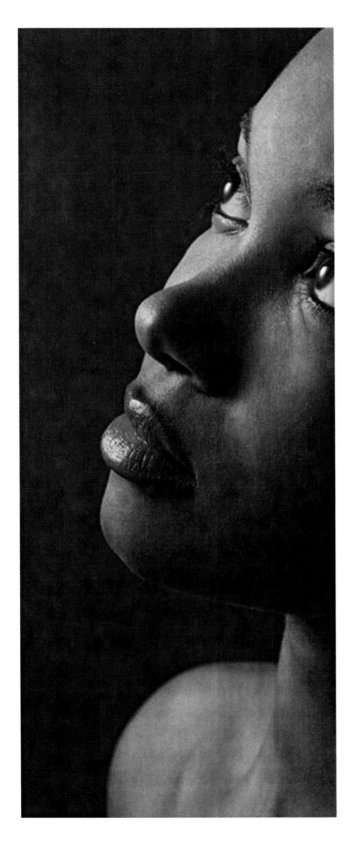

Uterine fibroids are estrogen-dependent tumors that are made worse by toxins in the environment, food and household products, such as dioxins and xenoestrogens. FibroidClear is designed to rebalance estrogen levels, and provide you with ingredients that reduce fibroids in size, and ease your symptoms.

FibroidClear

FibroidClear is a formulation of organic and wildcrafted herbs designed to:

- Naturally reduce the estrogen excess that causes fibroids to grow

- Shrink benign tumors such as fibroids

- Prevent further growth of uterine fibroids naturally

- Reduce blood clotting and control excessive menstrual bleeding

- Raise progesterone levels to help shrink fibroids and ease menstruation

- Reduce the symptoms of Pre Menstrual Tension

- Regulate the menstrual cycle and balance hormones

- Strengthen and tone the uterine muscles, and reduce cramps and spasms

- Assist the body in replenishing nutrients lost due to heavy menstruation

- Reduce tiredness and anemia caused by heavy periods

- Keep the tissues that surround the reproductive organs healthy

- Manage the energy levels throughout the month

- Reduce fluid retention, bloating and inflammation

- Strengthen the immune system and keep the uterus free of infection

Ingredients

Chaste Tree

Chaste Tree suppresses the over-production of estrogen and is widely used to balance hormones and treat premenstrual symptoms. Many double-blind placebo-controlled studies have proven its effectiveness, for example, the Institute for Health Care and Science in Germany found that 52% of women taking this supplement experienced significant improvements in menstrual symptoms such as bloating, headaches and irritability.

Chaste Tree also reduces estrogen levels while elevating progesterone levels, and has strong anti inflammatory, antibacterial and antifungal effects which helps the body to shrink fibroids.

Red Raspberry

Red Raspberry is used to control excessive menstrual bleeding and strengthens and tones the uterine muscles. Red Raspberry is very helpful in supporting the body return the reproductive organs into balance. It's anti inflammatory and anti nausea effects makes Red Raspberry a powerful herb for menstrual problems.

Red Raspberry is a rich source of nutrients, including Calcium, Magnesium, Iron, Potassium, Phosphorus, and Vitamins A, B, C and E. Also rich in tocopherols, carotenoids, and natural antioxidants, Numerous studies indicate that Red Raspberry helps to manage blood sugar levels, helping you keep your energy levels high throughout the month.

Motherwort

Motherwort is used world-wide for a range of menstrual and reproductive problems. It contains leonurine which relaxes the smooth muscles of the uterus, preventing cramping, and reducing menstrual pain.

Motherwort regulates menstruation, reduces cramping, balances hormones and reduces heavy bleeding, especially when mixed with Red Raspberry.

Siberian Ginseng

Siberian Ginseng has been used for over 4,000 in Chinese Medicine years to combat anemia caused by heavy bleeding, and maintain the energy levels. Like Red Raspberry, Siberian Ginseng helps manage blood sugar levels, preventing energy slumps throughout the month.

Siberian Ginseng contains properties that support the adrenal glands, and enables the body to cope with physical and mental stress. It also reduces blood clotting, especially when mixed with Red Clover.

Red Clover

Red Clover's daidzein and genistein compounds in are recognized by The National Cancer Institute to have anti-tumor properties. It is also a well-known blood cleansing herb, and supports detoxification, and it helps the liver to detoxify excess estrogen - the main cause of fibroids.

Red Clover has antispamodic and sedative qualities, calming the uterus, adn its as its phytoestrogens (plant estrogens) help balance the body's natural estrogen levels and regulate the menstrual cycle.

Rich in nutrients, it helps to replenish the body after many months of heavy bleeding. Red Clover contains tocopheral (Vitamin E), protein, and salicylates and coumarins, which reduce blood clotting.

Licorice Root

Licorice Root is used to treat fluid retention, helping with bloating and weight gain during menstruation. The Mjölbolsta Hospital found people taking Licorice over 8 weeks retained less water and normalized blood pressure levels.

Licorice Root is also used to calm the digestion, and when combined with Red Clover, supports the liver in breaking down excess estrogen.

Burdock Root

Burdock Root is another blood purifying herb, used to support the liver and detoxify excess estrogen and xenoestrogens.

It also has diuretic qualities, which help the body get rid of retained water, reducing bloating and swelling. Its anti-inflammatory properties also assist in shrinking fibroids in size.

Burdock Root is rich in Arctigenin, which inhibits the growth of tumors.

Goldenseal

Goldenseal helps to keep the uterus free of inflammation and infection. It has been used for hundreds of years by Native Americans for skin problems. It is also used to maintain the health of mucus membranes - the tissue surrounding the internal genitals.

The berberine in Goldenseal is antibacterial and anti-viral, which helps the body fight infection and strengthens the immune system, especially when combined with

Echinacea.

Echinacea has been used for over 400 years as a general cure-all. Recent studies suggest that Echinacea enhances the immune system, reduces inflammation and relieves pain.

For example, the Phytomedicine Journal reported a double-blind study in which subjects given Echinacea increased the functioning of the immune system by 120%. Additionally researchers in Germany found that large doses of echinacea healed wounds completely in just 7 days.

Echinacea has also been used to control benign growths and tumors such as fibroids.

How To Use FibroidClear

Take one capsule of FibroidClear with a meal, three times a day.

Frequently Asked Questions

Question: Will I notice changes in my cycle?

Answer: Since FibroidClear works on balancing the hormones, changes in your menstrual cycle are likely, as it shifts to a

lighter flow and a shorter duration of bleeding. Please allow 2-3 months for your new cycle to work itself out.

Question: My fibroids are extremely large. What do you recommend?

Answer: Our most powerful recommendation would be for you to do a body cleanse with the Body Cleanse Kit, in order to detoxify the chemical toxins that cause fibroids to grow, and to strengthen the organs responsible for recycling hormones and neutralizing toxins.

To prolong the effects and to support your body with the nutrients required to strengthen the organs, detoxify and heal the uterus, take AlkaGreens Plus 1-3 times a day. AlkaGreens Plus can also provide you with energy if you are feeling run down as a result of anemia or heavy periods.

Question: How long before I start to see results?

Answer: While every woman is biologically different, we find that most will get results after taking the herbal remedies for 3-4 months.

There are other factors that will accelerate the rate at which you get results:

- Doing a body cleanse with an organic body cleanse kit

- Eating organic food

- Making lifestyle changes, such as cutting out major sources of xenoestrogens

- Taking a food based nutrient supplement like AlkaGreens Plus

We find that women who make a large effort to make changes to their health get faster, and longer lasting results.

Question: I want to get pregnant but I have fibroids, Should I take FertilPlus For Women at the same time as taking FibroidClear?

Answer: Your best course of action would be to do a 4-month Fibroid Shrinking Program, which can reduce your fibroids in size, while rebalancing your hormone levels. Once your fibroids have shrunk, you can switch to taking FertilPlus for Women.

Question: I have just found out that I am pregnant, and I want to keep taking FibroidClear. Do you advise this?

If you are pregnant we do not recommend you take herbal products to shrink fibroids.

However, our pregnant customers are safely taking AlkaGreens Plus, which helps the body detox the substances that cause fibroids, while providing nutrition for both mother and baby.

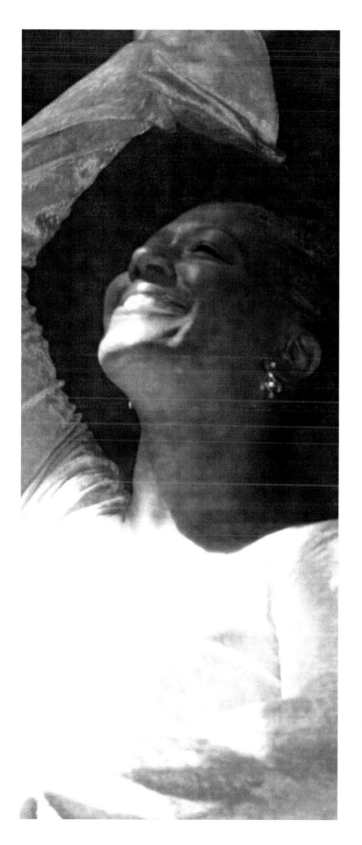

If you are looking for a complete solution

Fibroid Shrinking Kit

We have put together what we have found works best for women with large fibroids, or women with fibroids who want to conceive:

1. Body cleanse kit, consisting of:

   - Colon Cleansing Kit

   - Liver Cleansing Kit

   - Kidney Cleansing Kit

   - Toxin Cleansing Kit

2. 4 month supply of FibroidClear

3. 4 month supply of AlkaGreens Plus

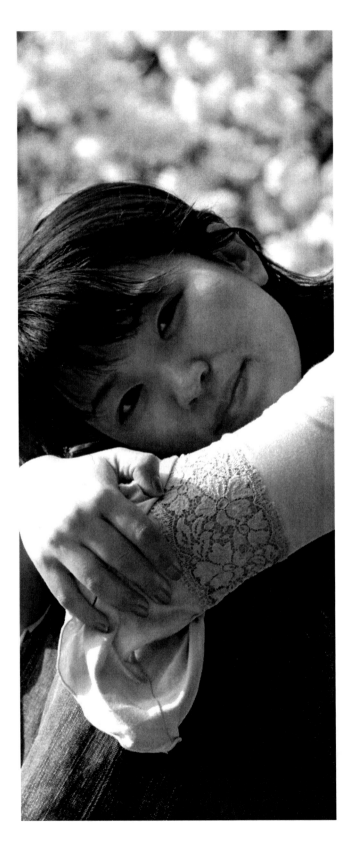

Endometriosis is a debilitation condition in which the cells that line the uterus grow in outside the uterus, for example, the vagina, cervix and colon, causing severe pain, reduced fertility and a reduced quality of life.

EndoClear

EndoClear contains herbs scientifically proven – by doctors, scientists and medical researchers – to clear endometrial growths, and reduce the symptoms of endometriosis rapidly. EndoClear is designed to:

- Balance estrogen levels - estrogen causes endometriosis symptoms to worsen

- Give fast relief from the symptoms of endometriosis and is scientifically proven to decrease the symptoms of PMS in 93% of women

- Relax the smooth muscle tissue of the uterus, and reduce uterine spasms and cramping

- Inhibit endometrial growths from forming, and help to keep existing endometrial growths under control

- Reduce inflammation and pain

- Boost the immune system and reduce infection, assisting the white blood cells to get rid of stray endometrial cells

- Reduce excess bleeding and reduce ruptures of endometrial growths, and controls bleeding and spotting in between periods

- Reduce the symptoms of irritable bowel syndrome

- Help to control stress and anxiety

- Boost energy levels

Ingredients

Chasteberry

Chasteberry has been used for centuries in Western and Chinese Medicine to treat gynaecological conditions, including endometriosis. Combined with Dong Quai it makes a powerful treatment for balancing hormones and reducing the pain of endometriosis. When Chasteberry is combined with Wild Yam it relaxes the uterus, reducing cramps and spasms.

It's approved by the German Commission E for family physicians and gynecologists to use for menstrual conditions. In fact, a German study reported that 52% of women taking this herbs reported a complete reduction in symptoms. Another German study reported 93% of women noticing a significant decrease in PMS symptoms.

Chasteberry is rich in essential oils and flavinoids. It works by stimulating the body to decrease estrogen levels and increase progesterone levels, leading to decreased occurrences in endometriosis.

Dong Quai

Dong Quai is also used in Traditional Chinese Medicine to treat female reproductive health complaints, including endometriosis, fibroids, PMS and infertility.

A Taiwan medical study found that Dong Quai inhibited tumor growth by 30%. Chinese Researchers found that the polysaccharides in Dong Quai improved the immune system by activating the T cells.

NYU School of Medicine found that the water-soluble components in Dong Quai had an anti inflammatory and antibacterial effect.

The Fourth Military Medical University in China found that Dong Quai prevented the blood cells from clumping together and improved the circulation of blood.

Wild Yam

Wild Yam has been used in the West since the 18th century to treat menstrual cramps and other gynaecological condition such as endometriosis. It is rich in diosgenin, a substance used by the body to create progesterone.

Wild Yam is effective for balancing estrogen levels, and researchers in Taiwan found that its phytoestrogens (a weak form of plant estrogen) bind to estrogen receptors in the body, replacing the stronger and more dangerous forms of estrogen such as xenoestrogens.

Psychiatrists in China reported that Wild Yam reduces anxiety levels, and its anti inflammatory and anti spasmodic effects are excellent for maintaining uterine health. When combined with Chasteberry and Cramp bark, Wild Yam is a powerful natural remedy for immediate relief from endo symptoms.

Cramp Bark

Cramp bark has been used for hundreds of years by Native Americans to treat pains and muscular cramping in the body. It is used to relax muscles, and is particularly effective on the smooth muscle cells of the uterus.

It also has anti-inflammatory effects and calms and soothes the nerves, reduces excess bleeding and provides great relief for dysmenorrhea.

It also has wonderful effects on irritable bowel syndrome and researchers at Lviv National Medical University, Ukraine found that it was an effective treatment for gastrointestinal damage.

Ginger

Ginger has been used for thousands of years in Chinese Medicine to reduce nausea, reduce pain, treat digestive complaints and to boost energy levels. It has been effectively used in India to improve allergic response, due to its anti inflammatory effects.

Doctors in Bangkok found that Ginger reduced nausea and vomiting in pregnant patients, while Scientists in Pakistan found that Ginger enhanced the travel of food through the intestine.

It is also good for preventing endometrial growths, as Doctors at the China Medical University, Taiwan proved that Ginger prevented blood cells from aggregating. Researchers at Seoul National University also found that the gingerol and vanilloids in ginger had anti-tumor properties.

Echinacea

Echinacea helps combat endometriosis by boosting the immune system, helping the body to get rid of stray endometrial cells, and by reducing inflammation and infections associated with endometriosis.

Echinacea works by enhancing immune response, encouraging the white blood cells to destroy foreign substances. Australian researchers found it is also a powerful antioxidant.

The beneficial effects of Echinacea on the immune system are well documented; one study carried out at Karl Franzens University, Austria demonstrated the effect the herb had on the innate and adaptive immune system. Research at the National College of Naturopathic Medicine, Portland, Oregon also confirms this fact.

Echinacea is used to improve conditions caused by imbalances in the immune system. The University of Marche in Italy found the herb effective and safe for treating patients suffering from an autoimmune condition.

Goldenseal

Goldenseal has been used for hundreds of years by Native Americans for its anti bacterial and anti-inflammatory properties.

It is particularly useful in endometriosis as it relaxes the uterine muscles, helps to reduce excessive bleeding, including bleeding in between periods, hemorrhages, and ruptures of endometrial growths.

Its anti-bacterial effects were documented by the University of Illionois, and the berberine in Goldenseal, along with Echinacea are both effective for clearing the body of infections and inflammations that cause painful endometriosis symptoms.

Calendula Flower

Calendula is very effective for boosting the immune system (especially when combined with Echinacea), repairing connective tissue, and improving the circulation of blood. It is also a natural pain killer.

Calendula is used to treat wounds, and is rich in plant antioxidants which protect the body from the free radicals that damage cells. It also has anti-inflammatory, antibacterial and anti-viral properties, which are very useful for keeping endometrial growths under control.

This is a great herb to have in any formula, as it improves the delivery of other herbs into the blood and lymphatic system, giving faster and more efficient benefits.

How To Take EndoClear

Take one capsule, three times a day with meals.

For fast, effective results, combine EndoClear with a Body Cleanse, and AlkaGreens Plus.

Frequently Asked Questions

Question: I want to get pregnant - should I take EndoClear or FertilPlus For Women?

Answer: We recommend you focus on getting the endometriosis under control first. Some women find that combining the Body Cleansing Kit, AlkaGreens Plus and EndoClear is enough to help them conceive.

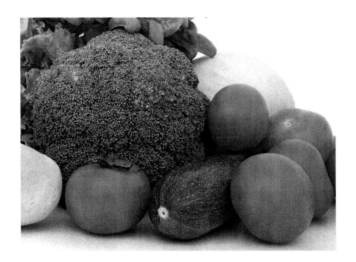

Superfoods are the ideal addition to any Natural Health Program, as they provide your body with essential nutrients recommended for the body to heal itself.

What's more, many superfoods are easy to digest, which can mean rapid results.

Superfoods

Why Do We Need Superfoods?

A superfood is a food that is rich in nutrients, low in calories and provides an extensive range of health benefits. One of the most important features of a superfood is that it should be easy to digest and assimilate.

The majority of superfoods are actually fruits and vegetables. It's a well-known fact that eating fruits and vegetables are essential for leading a healthy life, and preventing the onset of diseases. Even the US Government states:

> ***Most fruits and vegetables are naturally low in calories and provide essential nutrients and dietary fiber. They may also play a role in preventing certain chronic diseases.***

When compared to people who eat only small amounts of fruits and vegetables, those who eat more generous amounts, as part of a healthy diet, tend to have reduced risk of chronic diseases. These diseases include stroke, type 2 diabetes, some types of cancer, and perhaps cardiovascular disease and hypertension.

With many fruits and vegetables you buy from the stores being sprayed with pesticides, and grown in contaminated soil, it is difficult to know what to do in order to stay healthy.

Of course, organic fruits and vegetables are an excellent alternative to the commercial and contaminated produce available in the stores. However, it is difficult to stick to an organic regimen if you are eating out, do not prepare your own food, or do not have access to your own kitchen.

Many people do not have the time to eat the wide variety of fruits and vegetables recommended by governments and health authorities, so a SuperFood supplement makes a convenient alternative to anyone who is too busy, or unable to obtain organic fruits and vegetables.

Why Can Superfoods Replace Multivitamin Supplements?

If you are currently taking a multivitamin and mineral supplement purchased from a supermarket, or a local drug store, you may be unaware that the majority of what you are taking is not digestible by the human body.

For example, a study carried out in Salt Lake City found over 50 gallons of undigested vitamin and mineral pills in the sewers every month. Similar results were found in Tacoma, Washington where over 50,000 pounds of undigested vitamin and mineral pills are filtered out of the sewers every year.

This is because the body cannot digest synthetic vitamins and mineral supplements . Synthetic supplements are those developed in laboratories to mimic the molecular structure of natural vitamins, and are usually made from byproducts of the petroleum industry. They often contain preservatives, binders, and fillers to make them look attractive and have a longer shelf life.

Although these synthetic vitamins appear similar to the natural vitamins, it is difficult for the digestive system to break them down and absorb, and the small amount that is absorbed is not recognized by the cells, so are rejected at a cellular level, and end up excreted by the body in the form of urine and feces.

Antioxidants

Antioxidants are unfortunately, a necessity in the world in which we live. This is due to the dramatic increase in free radicals we're exposed to on a daily basis. Free radicals are created from air pollution, exhaust fumes, cigarette smoke, chemical byproducts, toxic waste, pesticides, electromagnetic radiation from cellphones, masts, laptops and computer screens, ultraviolet light and highly processed commercial foods and trans fats.

A free radical is a molecule that has lost one of its electrons and attempts to restore its balance by taking an electron from one a molecule that belongs to one of your cells. Free radicals can alter the DNA of cells, erode cell membranes, change the molecular structure of cells and destroy enzymes and proteins required for essential bodily functions. These harmful changes accelerate aging and leave us susceptible to diseases such a heart disease and cancer.

Free radicals are also partially responsible for premature aging, and can accelerate the aging of the female reproductive system, leaving younger women incapable of conceiving, and damage eggs, embryos and the placenta, making them incapable of sustaining a healthy pregnancy to full term.

Free radicals also affect male fertility, as they damage sperm, preventing them from being motile and in some cases, damaging sperm cells to the extent they are unable to penetrate the egg. In fact, studies have linked high free radical content in semen with low sperm counts, abnormal sperm morphology, poor sperm motility and low sperm vitality.

Antioxidants are compounds that scavenge free radicals and stop them from damaging cells, by providing them with electrons, so they do not need to damage your cells. Antioxidants also help your body to repair free-radical damaged cells as they provide additional electrons and nutrients required for rebuilding cells, reducing inflammation and reversing the aging of cells and tissues.

You can get antioxidants from organic fruit and vegetables, and many researchers suggest eating 7 to 9 portions of fruits and vegetables a day in order to get the antioxidants required to reverse aging. This may not be affordable or feasible for many people, as access to a wide variety of organic produce can be limited at work, or there is a limited time or budget for purchasing and preparing organic fruit and vegetables.

Antioxidant supplements, such as AntioxiPlus, containing ground forms of antioxidant fruits and vegetables are an excellent alternative that ensures you consume enough antioxidants to reverse the damage done by free radicals.

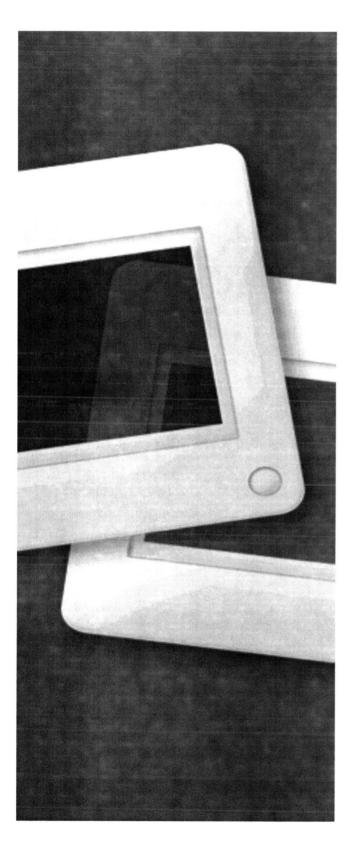

AlkaGreens Plus provides the body with nutrient-rich superfoods required for gentle detoxification, and creates an internal environment that supports healthy cells, and one in which yeast, fungus and bacteria cannot survive.

AlkaGreens Plus

The benefits of CraveEx are below:

- Boosting your energy levels without adding calories

- Balancing blood sugar levels, managing cravings and appetite

- Accelerating weight loss and assisting in the management of a healthy weight

- Boosts the immune system

- Strengthens the endocrine system and balances hormone levels

- Providing support to the adrenal glands and sympathetic nervous system, increasing your ability to deal with stress

- Assists in athletic performance, by providing nutrients required for exercise

- Provides the brain with fuel for increased concentration and improved memory

- Completely safe to take during pregnancy, and provides both the mother and fetus with nutrients required for a healthy pregnancy

The ingredients in AlkaGreens Plus can help you detoxify your blood and remove toxins and heavy metals, as they bind their molecular structures, so they can be safely removed by the body.

They also help reduce dioxin levels in the blood, and being rich in chlorophyll, they are powerful blood cleansers that purify the blood, assist in detoxification and help the cells to regenerate

They are rich in Gamma Linoliec Acid, which is an essential fatty acid that can help balance the hormones..

These foods also support the liver and digestive system, as they are rich in amino acids and contain polysaccharides such as beta glucan, which can help repair damaged cells and increase the efficiency of the liver in neutralizing toxins.

Ingredients

Hawaiian Spirulina

Hawaiian Spirulina is rich in beta carotene, vitamin B12, and a variety of minerals and essential amino acids. This species of spirulina has anti tumor properties, and contains Gamma Linolenic Acid, which reduces inflammation and can combat PMS.

Chlorella

Chlorella is an enzyme rich, easy to digest food is an excellent source of a variety of vitamins, minerals, essential fatty acids, and amino acids. It is a rich source of the blood-cleansing photochemical chlorophyll, and is a powerful detoxer as it binds with heavy metals, polychlorobinphenyls, and pesticides.

Purple Dulse Seaweed

Purple Dulse Seaweed is one of the richest sources of plant-based minerals, and is a powerful detoxifier of the blood, lymphatic system and can lower cholesterol levels. Dulse also boasts anti tumor properties, and is rich in natural iodine, which supports the thyroid.

Wheat Grass

Wheat Grass contains more nutrients per pound than most vegetables, and is rich in enzymes, chlorophyll, and the antioxidant enzyme Superoxide Dismutase, which converts dangerous free radicals into harmless compounds.

Spinach Leaf

Amongst its many health benefits, spinach contains quercetin, which reduces inflammation, and it is rich in flavinoids and antioxidants. Spinach contains a compound called neoxanthin, which can cause some tumor cells to self-destruct. It builds the blood, because it is naturally rich in iron.

Alfalfa Grass

Alfalfa Grass contains a wide variety of vitamins, minerals and other phytonutrients, and is rich in enzymes that enables the digestion of protein and carbohydrates.

Barley Grass

Barley Grass is an enzyme rich edible grass, which aids the digestion, supports the metabolism, reduces inflammation and boosts the immune system. It is rich in phytochemicals that detoxify the blood and reduce the effects of toxins and carcinogens on the body.

Rose Hips

Rose hips is the richest plant source of vitamin C, and contains essential fatty acids, which help balance the hormones and reduce inflammation, antioxidants, and iron, which supports women suffering heavy periods and anemia due to fibroids.

Orange Peel

Orange peel is rich in limonoids and vitamin C, and has over 170 tumor-fighting phytochemicals and 60 flavoinoids. It is rich in hesperidin, a flavinoid that strengthens the capillaries, and it has anti inflammatory properties.

Lemon Peel

Lemon peel is beneficial for the digestion, liver functioning and bile production, and are a great source of vitamin C. Lemons are also rich in limonene, which protect against cancer, and tumor formation. It can help convert fat into energy, so assists weight loss.

Astragalus Root

Astragalus root protects the liver, kidneys and urinary system, and supports the immune system. It is rich in antioxidants, and has anti-inflammatory properties. It also provides a gentle energy boost, while strengthening the body from disease.

Nettle Leaf

Nettle leaf - helps the body maintain a healthy electrolyte balance, reduces inflammation and assists detoxification of the blood. It can build the blood and is a common alternative remedy for anemia.

Beet Root

Beet root is a powerful blood builder as it is rich in iron and other vitamins and minerals required to support healthy red blood cells. It also contains phytochemicals that support healthy digestion, and a healthy liver and colon.

How To Take AlkaGreens Plus

Mix two level tablespoons (one scoop) of AlkaGreens Plus in 16oz (450ml) of fruit or vegetable juice and drink. Alternatively, mix 8 oz oz (225ml) ounces of pure water, 8 oz oz (225ml) of fruit juice, ½ cup of fresh fruit and two level tablespoons (one scoop) of AlkaGreens Plus..

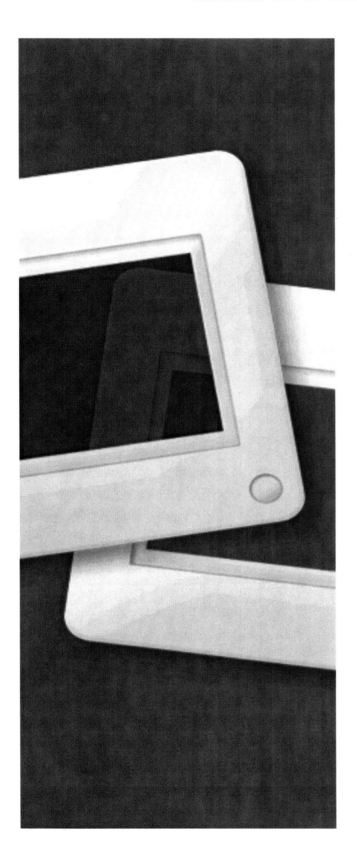

AntioxiPlus is a blend of antioxidant-rich superfoods that give the body natural protection from free radical damage.

AntioxiPlus

Antioxiplus is an organic and wildcrafted supplement recommended to help reverse aging of cells, and protect against free radicals and free radical damage. It contains many of the most potent antioxidant fruits, and is in a ground form, which makes it easy for your body to digest and assimilate.

Its benefits include:

- Improving the quality of eggs and protecting them from DNA damage

- Protecting the reproductive organs from aging and helping mature mothers to lower their reproductive age

- Creating healthy sperm with fewer defects, and reducing the risk of birth defects

- Helping the male reproductive system to create well-formed motile sperm

- Reducing the number of dead or damaged sperm

- Reducing inflammation and healing the repair of tissues, which is helpful for women with reproductive disorders

- Slowing down the signs of aging and keeping the skin looking young

- Supporting the immune system and helping the body fight disease and infection

Ingredients

Arcerola Cherries

Cherries contain anti-inflammatory compounds called anthocyanins, and are rich in quercetin, which reduces inflammation; ellagic acid, which is a naturally anti-cancer compound that causes apoptosis (cell death) of cancer cells while keeping normal cells healthy; and perillyl alcohol, which inhibits the growth of tumors.

Blueberry powder

Blueberries have the highest Oxygen Radical Absorbance Capacity (ORAC) values of all the foods in the world, which means it's the world's most powerful antioxidant fruit.

Blueberries have been noted by scientists to fight cancer, as they contain a compound that inhibit a cancer-promoting enzyme. They contain pterostilbene, which lowers blood lipid levels and prevents plaque from forming in the arteries.

Grape seed and Grape skin

Grapes are rich in reservatrol a compound that attacks microorganisms that cause disease, and has natural antimutagenic properties that stop cells from mutating and becoming cancerous.

Reservatrol is also a powerful antioxidant that has anti-aging properties and extends the life-span of cells.

Grape seeds and skin contain oligomeric proantho cyanins (OPCs), which are antioxidants more than vitamin C and E, and protect the body from damage from environmental pollution and stress. OPCs can reverse the effect of high cholesterol and protect the heart and lower LDL cholesterol. They are also a natural antihistimine and reduce allergic reactions and inflammation.

Green Tea

The polyphenols in tea can halve free radical cellular damage, neutralize enzymes for tumor growth and deactivate cancer promoters.

Green tea is rich in catechins, especially EGCG, which has numerous anti-cancer benefits. It lowers fibrinogen, a substance that causes clots and increases the risk of strokes and thrombosis, and reduces the risk of developing coronary artery disease.

The Nippon Medical School found it was good for weight loss, as it stimulates the metabolism and balances blood sugar.

It also contains theanine, which encourages the release of dopamine and GABA, and is rich in antioxidants that prevent degenerative disease.

Maca

Maca contains B vitamins, and a wide range of minerals, including calcium, iron, manganese, magnesium, phosphorous, selenium and zinc, It also contains plant compounds scientifically proven in scientific to support the endocrine system, which includes the male and female reproductive.

Mangosteen

Mangoseen are rich in antioxidants called xanthones, which help to maintain a healthy immune system and have natural anti-inflammatory, anti-viral and antibiotic effects. Xanthones are also beneficial for cardiovascular and joint health.

They also have an Oxygen Radical Absorbance Capacity over 14 times that of red raspberries.

Orange Powder

Orange skin is rich in limonoids and vitamin C, and has anti-viral, antibacterial, anti-fungal, antimalarial and antineoplasctic qualities. Organe has over 170 anticancer phytochemicals and 60 flavoinoids. It is rich in hesperidin, a flavinoid that strengthens the capillaries, and it protects the heart as it is anti inflammatory, anti allergenic, vasoprotective and anti-carcinogenic.

It is also rich in compounds that lower the risk of stroke, high blood pressure and lowers Lower Density Lipoprotein cholesterol (bad cholesterol), while raising High Density Liportein cholesterol (good cholesterol).

In addition, organges are rich in potassium, which lowers blood pressure, pectin, which lowers cholesterol, and folate, which lowers homocysteine. It contains calcium, in a format that is beneficial for your bones and teeth, and is rich in the cartenoid betacryptoxanthin, which protects the heart.

Papaya

Papaya is a great source of digestive enzymes and is rich in papain, potassium, fiber, calcium, folate, vitamin C, beta carotene, letein and zeaxanthin, which all support the immune system.

Pineapple

Pineapples are rich in bromelain, an enzyme that speeds up th healing of wounds, aids the digestion of proteins, reduces inflammation and bruising, and prevents the aggregation of platelets.

They are also rich in manganese, which is beneficial for healthy bones, cartilage and skin, and activates an antioxidant enzyme called super oxide dismutase (SOD), and balances blood sugar levels. Pineapples are also a good source of vitamins C and potassium.

Pomegranate seed

Pomegranates contain a higher concentration of flavinoids than grapes, and have powerful antioxidant effects, antimicrobial and anti-cancer activity.

It contains compounds that inhibit LDL oxidization, improves cardiovascular health and reduces plaque in the arteries.

Raspberry

Raspberries are one of the most high fiber fruits in the world, and a rich source of vitamins C and K, calcium, magnesium, phosphorus and potassium. They are one of the richest sources of anthocynins, which reduce pain and inflammation

Most importantly, they are the best source of ellagic acid, which inhibits the growth of tumors and causes apoptosis in cancer cells (cell death), and has anti-viral and antibacterial properties too.

Shiitake mushrooms

Shiitake mushrooms are valued in Asian cultures for their medicinal effects. They contain all 8 of the essential amino acids and are rich in linoleic acid. Shiitake mushrooms are rich in eritadenine, a compound that lowers cholesterol, and is rich enzymes. Shiitake mushrooms also contain high levels of betaglucons, which boost the immune system, and in particular, Betaglucan 1.3, which increases the activity of macrophages – cells that scavenge debris and foreign microbes.

Shiitake mushrooms are also ideal for detoxification as they absorb toxins and help the body to eliminate them safely.

Tumeric

Turmeric contains circumin, which reduces inflammation by lowering histamine levels. It has anti-tumor properties and inhibits cancer cell growth.

It protects the body from accumulating cholesterol, and it protects your eyes from cataracts

It is great for liver health, as it lowers elevated liver enzymes.

Wolfberry

Also known as Goji Berries, wolfberries contain 18 amino acids, 21 trace minerals and are rich in vitamin C, cartenoids and are high in fiber. The polysaccharides of wofberries are powerful antioxidants that boost the immune system and reduce tumor size.

How To Take AntioxiPlus

Take 3 capsules with breakfast each day.

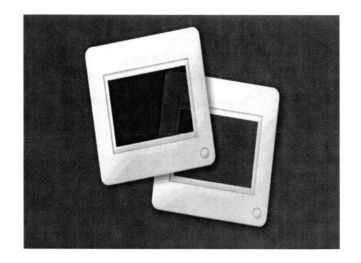

Recent developments in brain technologies have enabled people to bring about significant health and lifestyle changes with little time and expense. Quantum Subliminals bypass the subliminal mind, allowing you to design your life and behaviors according to your wishes.

Subliminals

Subliminal Brain Technology

Quantum Subliminals is a powerful technology that bypasses the conscious mind, and reaches the brains subconscious levels in order to produce changes.

Subliminal messages are those that reach the subconscious mind, by passing through conscious human perception.

Affirmations Do Not Work

While many of these techniques help in areas in which you already excel, they cannot produce changes you want in your areas of weakness, as these positive messages are over-ruled by a skeptical conscious mind and negative self-beliefs.

Unlike positive affirmations and many forms of hypnosis, Quantum Subliminals allow positive, life-changing messages to reach the subconscious mind, and rescript behavior patterns without resistance of the conscious mind.

What Are Quantum Subliminals?

Quantum Subliminals come in the form of a regular compact disk, and provide you with positive messages that bypass your conscious brain. Quantum Subliminals combines the technologies of binaural beats, silent subliminals and Neuro Linguistic Programming to exact powerful positive changes to your thoughts and behaviors.

The binaural beats gently alter the frequencies of your brain waves from the Beta range (normally associated with the stress of every day life), down to the Alpha range, which is associated with alert relaxation.

After your brain has adjusted to the Alpha range, you will be gently guided to the deep meditative Theta frequencies, allowing you to access a calm and tranquillity only achievable through years of meditation or brain-wave technology audios such as Quantum Relaxation

These messages are inaudible to the conscious brain, and are masked by sounds from nature, such as waterfalls, or rain.

How To Use Quantum Subliminals

Quantum Subliminals are very easy to use, as you do not need to visualize, focus on a voice or repeat any affirmations to achieve the benefits. Simply close your eyes and let the brain-wave audio technology do the work.

All you need is a pair of headphones, so that the binaural beats can do their work. You can listen to them while relaxing in a comfortable chair, before you go to sleep, or even while sleeping. Some people prefer to listen to them in their sleep, as the audios can bring about a more restful sleep.

Available Titles

- Quantum Relaxation

Product Listing

AlkaGreens Plus

AlkaGreens Plus is a naturally balanced blend of organic superfoods, specifically formulated to supply natural food source vitamins, minerals, amino acids, enzymes and essential trace nutrients.

Price:

1 bottle of AlkaGreens Plus - $77

2 bottles of AlkaGreens Plus - $137 saving $17

3 bottles of AlkaGreens Plus - $197 saving $34

4 bottles of AlkaGreens Plus - $249 saving $59

Ingredients: Hawaiian Spirulina Blue-Green Algae, Chlorella broken cell Algae, Purple Dulse Seaweed, Wheat Grass, Spinach leaf, Alfalfa Grass, Barley Grass, Rose hips, Orange peel, Lemon peel, Astragalus root, Nettle leaf, Beet root

Quantity: 14 ounces (396 grams) bottle with scoop

Supply: 28 day supply (1 scoop a day)

AntioxiPlus

Antioxiplus is an organic and wildcrafted supplement recommended to help reverse aging of cells, and protect against free radicals and free radical damage. It contains many of the most potent antioxidant fruits, and is in a ground form, which makes it easy for your body to digest and assimilate.

Price:

1 bottle of AntioxiPlus - $77

2 bottles of AntioxiPlus - $137 saving $17

3 bottles of AntioxiPlus - $197 saving $34

4 bottles of AntioxiPlus - $249 saving $59

Ingredients: Maca, Raspberry, Pineapple, Green Tea, Arcerola cherry, Blueberry powder, Shiitake mushrooms, Orange Powder, Grape seed, Grape skin, Pomegranate seed, Papaya, Tumeric, Wolfberry, Mangosteen

Quantity: 100 Capsules (515mg each)

Supply: 1 Month

Blocked Fallopian Tubes Fast Start CD

Fast start CD for the blocked fallopian tubes kit that explains what you need to do in order to get started.

Price: 1 Blocked Fallopian Tube Fast Start CD - $77

Quantity: 1 Audio CD

Blocked Fallopian Tubes Book

This book details the 7-steps involved in unblocking your fallopian tubes, using herbal tampons and describes the massage process for opening up blocked fallopian tubes.

Price: 1 Blocked Fallopian Tube Book - $77

Quantity: 1 hardcopy book

Body Cleanse Book

Instruction booklet that gives step-by-step instructions on how to use the body cleansing and detoxification products, including the body cleanse kit.

Price: 1 Body Cleansing Book - $47

Quantity: 1 hardcopy book

CarboClear

CarboClear prevents carbohydrates and sugars from being broken down and absorbed by the body, and contains natural ingredients that help the body expel the undigested carbs.

Price: 1 bottle of Carboclear - $67

Ingredients: White kidney bean extract, fenugreek, cinnamon, American ginseng

Quantity: 100 capsules (535mg) each

Supply: 1 month

Chamomile Cleanse

The Chamomile Cleanse herbal douche should be used with herbal tampons to wash the pelvic organs of any remaining infection and debris loosened by the herbal tampons

Price: 1 pouch of Chammomile Cleanse - $67

Ingredients: Chamomile, Pau D\'Arco

Quantity: 4oz foil pouch

Supply: 3 Menstrual cycles

Colon D-Tox 1

Colon D-Tox 1 is a powerful herbal formula for cleansing the colon and restoring intestinal function to normal.

Price: 1 bottle of Colon D-Tox 1- $57

Ingredients: African bird pepper, Barberry root bark, Cape aloes, Cascara sagrada aged bar, Fennel seed, Garlic bulb, Ginger root, Senna herb

Quantity: 100 capsules (435mg each)

Supply: 20 days

Colon D-Tox 2

Colon D-Tox 2 contains natural herbs and substances that soothe the colon, while creating an adhesive layer that draws out impacted waste from the colon walls to ease out waste that causes toxicity inflammation, IBS or other bowel problems.

Price: 1 bottle of Colon D-Tox 2 - $57

Ingredients: Activated willow charcoal, Apple fruit pectin, flax seeds, Marshmallow root, Pharmaceutical grade bentonite clay, Psyllium seeds and husks, Slippery elm inner bark,

Quantity: 1 8oz (225 grams) bottle with scoop

Supply: 20 days

CraveEx

CraveEx is designed to help you curb your cravings for carbohydrates and sweet foods, while supporting your efforts in losing weight. CraveEx can be taken every day with meals, to help you beat the habit of eating unhealthy foods

Price: 1 bottle of CraveEx - $67

Ingredients: Gymnema leaf, Stevia extract, Licorice root, Dandelion root

Quantity: 100 capsules (355mg each)

Supply: 1 Month Supply

DidaClear

DidaClear contains herbs that kill yeast and fungal infections such as candida, oral thrush and genital thrush.

Price: 1 bottle of DidaClear - $67

Ingredients: Pau D'Arco, Garlic, Echinacea, Goldenseal, Chamomile, Barberry root, Oregano oil

Quantity: 100 Capsules (405mg each)

Supply: 1 Month Supply

EndoClear

Endoclear contains herbs scientifically proven – by doctors, scientists and medical researchers – to clear endometrial growths, and reduce the symptoms of endometriosis rapidly.

Price:

1 bottle of EndoClear - $67

2 bottles of EndoClear - $97 saving $37

3 bottles of EndoClear - $137 saving $64

4 bottles of EndoClear - $177 saving $71

Ingredients: Chasteberry, Dong Quai, Echinacea, Cramp Bark, Ginger Root, Wild Yam, Goldenseal, Calendula Flower

Quantity: 100 capsules (325mg each)

Supply: 1 Month Supply

Fallopen Herbal Tampon Mix

Fallopen herbal tampon mix is a blend of organic and wildcrafted herbs for unblocking fallopian tubes. (It only includes the herbal mix, not the tampons, which need to be purchased separately.)

Price: 1 pouch of Fallopen Herbal Tampon Mix - $97

Ingredients: Calendula, Goldenseal, Garlic, Red Clover, Corydalis Root, Astragalus Root, Dong Quai, Ligusticum

Quantity: 4oz Foil Pouch

Supply: 3 Menstrual Cycles

FalloClear

FalloClear is a herbal capsule designed for unblocking the fallopian tubes, by allowing the herbs to reach the fallopian tubes indirectly, via the digestive system. FalloClear should be used with the herbal tampons and douches.

Price: 1 bottle of FalloClear - $97

Ingredients: Goldenseal, Tribulus Terrestris , Dong Quai, Pineapple Juice Powder, Astragalus Root, Garlic, Chaste Tree, Green Tea

Quantity: 100 Capsules (445mg each)

Supply: 1 Month Supply

FertilPlus For Men

Natural herbal supplement to help increase male sperm count, sperm motility and sperm vitality. A 3 month supply is recommended for good results, as it takes men 90 days to create new sperm.

Price:

1 bottle of FertilPlus For Men - $67

2 bottles of FertilPlus For Men - $97 saving $37

3 bottles of FertilPlus For Men - $137 saving $64

4 bottles of FertilPlus For Men - $177 saving $71

Ingredients: Ginger, Horny Goat Weed, Maca, Muira Puama, Panax Ginseng, Sarsaparilla, Saw Palmetto

Quantity: 100 Capsules (435mg each)

Supply: 1 Month

FertilPlus For Women

A herbal blend that balances the hormones, regulates ovulation, menstruation and boosts fertility in women by up to 330%

Price:

1 bottle of FertilPlus For Women - $67

2 bottles of FertilPlus For Women - $97 saving $37

3 bottles of FertilPlus For Women - $137 saving $64

4 bottles of FertilPlus For Women - $177 saving $71

Ingredients: Black Cohosh, Chaste Tree, Dong Quai, Green tea leaves, Muira Puama, Siberian Ginseng

Quantity: 100 capsules (330mg each)

Supply: 1 Month Supply

Fertility Massage DVD NTSC

The purpose of this fertility massage is to improve the flow of blood, lymphatic fluid, oxygen and nutrients to the pelvic organs in order to unblock your fallopian tubes, strengthen the uterus, facilitate conception and promote a healthy, problem-free pregnancy.

Price: 1 Fertility Masage DVD - $97

Quantity: 1 Region-Free DVD (USA & Canada Only)

Fertility Massage DVD PAL

The purpose of this fertility massage is to improve the flow of blood, lymphatic fluid, oxygen and nutrients to the pelvic organs in order to unblock your fallopian tubes, strengthen the uterus, facilitate conception and promote a healthy, problem-free pregnancy.

Price: 1 Fertility Masage DVD - $97

Quantity: 1 Region-Free DVD (OUTSIDE USA & Canada)

Fertility Yoga DVD PAL

Fertility yoga consists of the asanas (or positions) that nourish the reproductive organs, endocrine system and brain, while unblocking the fallopian tubes, opening up the pelvic organs and gently exercising the uterus, ovaries and fallopian tubes.

Price: 1 Fertility Yoga DVD - $97

Quantity: 1 Region-Free DVD (OUTSIDE USA & Canada)

Fertility Yoga DVD NTSC

Fertility yoga consists of the asanas (or positions) that nourish the reproductive organs, endocrine system and brain, while unblocking the fallopian tubes, opening up the pelvic organs and gently exercising the uterus, ovaries and fallopian tubes.

Price: 1 Fertility Yoga DVD - $97

Quantity: 1 Region-Free DVD (USA & Canada Only)

Unit Price: $97

FibroidClear

FibroidClear is a formulation of organic and wildcrafted herbs designed to reduce fibroids in size, and relieve the symptoms of uterine fibroids, including heavy periods, menstrual cramps, and abdominal bloating.

Price:

1 bottle of FibroidClear - $67

2 bottles of FibroidClear - $97 saving $37

3 bottles of FibroidClear - $137 saving $64

4 bottles of FibroidClear - $177 saving $71

Ingredients: Chaste tree, Red raspberry, Motherwort, Siberian ginseng, Red clover, Licorice root, Burdock root, Goldenseal, Echinacea

Quantity: 100 Capsules (320mg each)

Supply: 1 Month Supply

Kidney D-Tox Capsules

Kidney D-Tox is a natural organic formula that helps to cleanse the kidneys, bladder and urinary system.

Price: 1 bottle of Kidney D-Tox Capsules - $57

Ingredients: Burdock root, Corn silk, Gravel root, Horsetail herb, Hydrangea root, Juniper berries, Marshmallow root, Uva ursi leaves

Quantity: 100 Capsules (410mg each)

Supply: 20 Days supply

Kidney D-Tox Tea

Kidney D-Tox is a natural organic tea that helps to cleanse the kidneys, bladder and urinary system.

Price: 1 pouch of Kidney D-Tox Tea - $67

Ingredients: Alfalfa herb, Echinacea, Goldenseal, Licorice root, Nettle leaf, Parsley root, Rosemary leaf, Wild yam

Quantity: 4oz Foil Pouch

Supply: 20 Day Supply

LipoClear

LipoClear is a natural fat-blocker supplement that prevents the absorption of dietary fats, and helps the body to dispose of dietary fat without storing it as body fat.

Price: 1 bottle of LipoClear - $67

Ingredients: Psyllium husks, Guar gum, Green tea, Cayenne

Quantity: 100 Capsules (530mg each)

Supply: 30 Day Supply

Unit Price: $67

Liver D-Tox Capsules

Liver D-Tox is a powerful herbal formula for detoxifying the liver and gallbladder, and supporting their optimal functioning.

Price: 1 bottle of Liver D-Tox Capsules - $57

Ingredients: Dandelion root, Garlic bulb, Ginger root, Milk thistle seed, Oregon grape root, Wormwood leaf

Quantity: 100 Capsules (435mg)

Supply: 20 Days Supply

Liver D-Tox Tea

Liver D-Tox tea is a great-tasting blend of herbs that gently cleanse the liver and gallbladder and support the liver cleansing process.

Price: 1 pouch of Liver D-Tox Tea - $57

Ingredients: Burdock root, Cinnamon bark, Dandelion root, Fennel seed, Green tea, Licorice root, Pau D\'Arco bark, Peppermint leaf

Quantity: 4oz Foil Pouch

Supply: 20 Day Supply

Metal D-Tox

Metal D-Tox can help you remove heavy metals from your body's tissues without side effects.

Price: 1 bottle of Metal D-Tox - $67

Ingredients: Cilantro (Coriander), Chlorella

Quantity: 100 Capsules (410mg each)

Supply: 20 Days Supply

Para D-Tox

Para D-Tox is a complete herbal solution for killing parasites, and contains ingredients that kill and expel over 100 known parasites.

Price: 1 bottle of Para D-Tox - $67

Ingredients: Black walnut, Cloves, Wormwood, Garlic, Ginger root, Cat\'s claw bark, Slippery elm

Quantity: 100 Capsules (390mg each)

Supply: 20 Days Supply

Quantum Subliminals CD

The Quantum Subliminals CD enables you to achieve deep levels of relaxation and regeneration, without meditating.

Available Titles:

- Free From Alcohol
- Free From Anger
- Free From Coffee
- Free From Depression
- Free From Pain
- Free From Procrastination
- Free From Smoking
- Free From Stress
- Quantum Confidence
- Quantum Fertility
- Quantum Healing
- Quantum Relaxation
- Quantum Sleep
- Quantum Speaking
- Quantum Success
- Quantum Thin
- Quantum Willpower

Price: 1 Quantum Subliminal CD - $77

Wulong-Oolong Tea

Wulong Oolong tea is a fat-burning, thermogenic tea that raises the metabolic rate and assists the body to burn stubborn body fat.

Price:

1 pouch of Wulong-Oolong Tea - $57

2 pouches of Wulong-Oolong Tea - $87 saving $27

3 pouches of Wulong-Oolong Tea - $117 saving $54

4 pouches of Wulong-Oolong Tea - $137 saving $91

5 pouches of Wulong-Oolong Tea - $157 saving $128

Ingredients: Oolong tea

Quantity: 4oz Foil Pouch

Supply: 1 Month Supply

Wulong Oolong Capsules

Wulong Oolong capsules contain the fat-burning, thermogenic tea that raises the metabolic rate and assists the body to burn stubborn body fat.

Price: 1 bottle of Wulong-Oolong capsules - $67

Ingredients: Oolong tea

Quantity: 100 Capsules (435mg each)

Supply: 30 Day Supply

Unit Price: $67

Kits

Mature Mother's Kit

A fertility-boosting kit, designed to help women over 35 to conceive.

Price:

3 Month Mature Mother's Kit for $898 saving $298

4 Month Mature Mother's Kit for $1052 saving $365

Contains:

- 3 or 4 month supply of FertilPlus For Women
- Body Cleansing Kit (for you to share) containing:
  - Colon Cleanse Kit

  - Liver Cleanse Kit
  - Kidney Cleanse Kit
  - FREE Toxin Cleanse Kit
- 3 or 4 month supply of AlkaGreens Plus
- 3 or 4 month supply of AntioxiPlus Capsules
- 1 Quantum Relaxation CD

Supply: 3 or 4 Months

Fibroid Shrinking Kit

Designed to help women with large fibroids, or those who want to get pregnant and have fibroids

Price:

3 Month Fibroid Shrinking Program for $624 saving $331

4 Month Fibroid Shrinking Program for $726 saving $373

Contains:

- 1 Body Cleanse Kit containing:
  - Colon Cleanse Kit
  - Liver Cleanse Kit
  - Kidney Cleanse Kit
  - FREE Toxin Cleanse Kit
- 3 or 4 month supply of AlkgaGreens Plus
- 3 or 4 Bottles of FibroidClear

Supply: 3 or 4 month supply

Ultra Nutrition Plus Kit

Price: 1 Ultra Nutrition Plus Kit for $97

Contains:

- 1 Month supply of AlkaGreens Plus

- 1 Month Supply of AnitoxiPlus

Supply: 1 Month

Body Cleanse Kit

Price: 1 Body Cleanse Kit for $297

Contains:

- Colon D-Tox 1

- Colon D-Tox 2

- Liver D-Tox Capsules

- Liver D-Tox Tea

- Kidney D-Tox Capsules

- Kidney D-Tox Tea

- Metal D-Tox

- Para D-Tox

Supply: Enough for 2 people to do a cleanse each

Blocked Fallopian Tube Kit

Price:

1 Blocked Fallopian Tube Kit (USA & Canada) for $497

1 Blocked Fallopian Tube Kit (Rest Of World) for $497

Contains:

- Blocked Fallopian Tubes Book

- Chamomile Cleanse Herbal Douche

- FalloClear Capsules

- Fertility Yoga DVD

- Quantum Relaxation CD

- Fallopen Herbal Tampon Mix

- Fertility Massage DVD

- Blocked Fallopian Tubes Fast Start CD

Supply: 3 Menstrual Cycles

How To Order Herbal Remedies

You can order online via our website: www.biotanicalhealth.com Or order via telephone:

USA: 1-800- 893-0319

UK: 020-8133-9730

Press 1 only if you are ready to order, and you will be forwarded to our Order Processing Center

2989235